Social Work and Community Care

Also by Malcolm Payne

Power, Authority and Responsibility in Social Services:
  Social Work in Area Teams*
Working in Teams*
Social Care in the Community*
Modern Social Work Theory: A Critical Introduction*
Linkages: Effective Networking in Social Care

*Also published by Macmillan

Social Work and Community Care

Malcolm Payne

Consultant Editor: Jo Campling

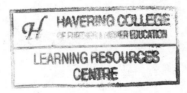

MACMILLAN

First published 1995 by
MACMILLAN PRESS LTD
Houndmills, Basingstoke, Hampshire RG21 2XS
and London
Companies and representatives
throughout the world

ISBN 0–333–60623–X
ISBN 0–333–60624–8

A catalogue record for this book is available
from the British Library.

10   9   8   7   6   5   4   3   2   1
04 03 02 01 00 99 98 97 96 95

Printed in Great Britain by
Mackays of Chatham PLC
Chatham, Kent

To Anne

Contents

List of Figures

List of Tables

Foreword and Acknowledgements

This book is concerned with the practice consequences of policy developments in community care following the *National Health Service and Community Care Act, 1990*. Social workers and their managers and policy-makers ought to see practice in the context of policy and organisation, and policy and organisation can only be understood as they are expressed through practice or at least the potential for it. It is unsatisfactory to explore policy without understanding the reality of the practice which will emanate from it. This view, which I hold very strongly, requires a better understanding of practice possibilities and options drawn from professional literature and understanding than we are accustomed to see in policy-oriented books. The corollary, that practice must come from a good understanding of the implementation of policy, is better appreciated. Nevertheless, in the social services of the early 1990s, policy-analysis related to practice seems to me to have two faults. It is either so critical as to be hostile to the innovation, or it derives from the government's own analysis of its policy, converted into practice and policy guidance and reinforced by selectively funded research. To be helpful, we must be constructively critical of the policy context of practice innovations. Yet we must try to understand what they mean for practice and how they might be implemented, even if at the same time we must be doubtful of their value.

This book also reflects my long-standing commitment to the exploration and understanding of practice. After the publication of the Barclay Report (1982), I wrote a book called *Social Care in the Community* (Payne, 1986a), in which I tried to analyse and describe the social work skills involved in 'social care planning', which was the Report's term for social work activities contrasted with 'counselling'. Skills such as enabling, negotiating, mobilising resources, networking and advocacy are as crucial in social work as the more therapeutic aspect of 'treatment' through counselling-type work, but are much less valued, less realised in accounts of social work practice and less taught than 'counselling'. The interest in anti-discriminatory work in the late 1980s and various advocacy movements have led to a strong development of empowerment and advocacy theory and writing, which was briefly presaged in my 1986 book.

Anxiety about policy issues such as community care plans, resource delegation and organisational and management reform seems to be leading to a neglect of the opportunities of the new community care system for doing more interesting and positive work for neglected groups of clients and their carers. Directors of social services have told me that training must concentrate on budgeting and management rather than on how to help people in the community in more imaginative ways. I hope this is just a characteristic of the setting-up phase of a new policy, but I fear that it reflects a longstanding attitude in the British social services that having good systems of organisation is the only thing needed for good services. Training and research funds so often follow this twisted view of the world, when the creativity of what social workers actually do in relationships with members of the public is just as important for the quality of services, if not more so. It seems that no amount of child care scandals has yet taught us that rigorous procedures, carefully implemented, have to be supplemented by putting sensitive, genuine, creative people into relationships with the public and supporting, training and enabling the use of their skills. To do this, we need a clear understanding of what professional practice can offer in a new policy context. That is what this book is about. It is based on my experience over the last ten years of the voluntary and community sector particularly in Liverpool and Manchester, and my period of development work in mental health with the Richmond Fellowship, and I am very grateful for the ideas and learning that I have gained from the people I have worked with.

I wish to acknowledge the technical help of Kathy Woods, of the Manchester Metropolitan University Computer Services Unit, and help and advice from my teaching colleagues Tony Sargeant and Simon Goodwin, practitioner colleague Jane Dalrymple and the ideas and experience of my 1992 masters class in care management.

Edgworth, Bolton   Malcolm Payne

Client, Consumer, User: A Note on Terminology

Many people are using the term 'service user' to refer to someone who receives services from social and health services, generally and in particular under community care legislation. This is intended to reflect a more empowered user with rights to control over the services provided, rather than someone who is the object of professional therapeutically-oriented service. I am a little cautious about this usage. For one thing, I think the use of language to denote something aspired to rather than actual creates a false impression, and I think that the 'empowered user' is not all that common in today's social and health services. Secondly, I do not wish to deny the value of professional, therapeutically-oriented service when it is desired, appropriate and produces a positive outcome. So, I do not want to avoid altogether the use of terms such as 'client' and 'patient' when it is relevant.

Similarly, some people are using the word 'consumer' because they want to promote the idea that users of services have the same rights as a customer in a shop to demand clear standards of service and rectification of bad service. This usage is designed to align service provision in the health and social services with general consumer movements in society. I am cautious about it for similar reasons to those that I have expressed about 'user'. Moreover, I think 'consumer' or, worse, 'customer' is a misuse when applied to social services where the 'client', to use the conventional term, is involved in a continuing relationship with the worker and participates actively in planning and implementing the service. 'Consumer' and 'customer' is also inappropriate in social and health services, in my view, because there should be rights to good service as citizens, rather than being called 'consumers' or 'customers' in some false analogy with customers in shops or banks.

Throughout this book, therefore, I have drawn a rather careful distinction between the circumstances in which I have used terminology about the people who are served by social and health services. Where I am referring to people who are the objects of traditional social work services, I have used the word 'client'; where they are receiving medical treatment or are in or being discharged from hospital, I have called them 'patients'and where they are genuinely receiving services in a position where they are or should be participating in the development and management of the service offered to them, I have used the word 'user'.

1

The Social Work Role in Community Care

The policy of community care is being actively implemented in British social services in the last years of the twentieth century and may come to fruition in the first years of the twenty-first. It is a culmination of a reaction against the social care policies of the nineteenth century, and an expression of many of the debates and ideas which are central to social services policies in the last half of the twentieth.

Looking at social work practice within community care means looking at policy in action. Discussing the analysis and description of practice options puts policy and organisation of services at the centre of practice debate. One reason for this is that, unusually for a social policy initiative, community care policy has *care management*, a major methodological and organisational reform, as part of its objectives. Another reason is that, unusually for a practice development, community care pratice is centrally about the effective use of resources, which is usually the province of management and politics.

Practice in community care is about resources, but not just how much funding government chooses to allocate to the social care needs of some of the most oppressed and disadvantaged groups in society. We must include all kinds of resources: personal, economic, social, political.

Social workers are a significant part of the provision of community care because they carry out three important roles, which form a linked pattern, shown in Figure 1.1.

● Through *care management,* they help clients clarify their needs

1

Figure 1.1. *The three community care roles of social work*

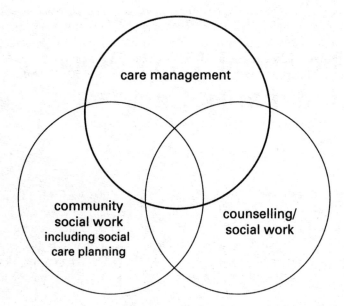

and make effective use of their own personal resources and community resources in meeting those needs.

- Through *community social work,* including the Barclay Report ideal of 'social care planning', they help develop community resources to provide for those in need.
- Through providing therapeutic *social work* as one of the services within community care, they help clients and the people around them deal with personal issues and difficulties and so help them to lead a more satisfying life which contributes to their family, community and social life.

Other groups of helpers, other occupations, share this work. Social workers are in a network of helping agencies and professions. Their skills are shared with those other agencies and occupations and with ordinary people in their everyday lives. Social workers, however, because of their training, skills and the focus of their work have these three special roles in helping others within the community care system. They can help clients and colleagues make the best of community resources both in personal and individual relationships and in more general social provision. The social work roles in community care, the policy developments and thinking that lie at its centre, and the skills involved in taking it on, are the main concern of this book. I argue, towards the end of this chapter, that social work has a particularly strong claim among occupational groups to offer useful skills, knowledge and training to community care.

Care management, counselling and social care

The Barclay Report (1982) distinguished two aspects of social work activities. Much social work uses direct relationships with workers – helping clients and the people around them change their relationships, so as to live their lives in a happier, more satisfying way, and to manage their lives more efficiently. The Barclay Report (1982) calls this 'counselling', and any work with a member of the public in providing caring services will inevitably contain elements of direct work of this kind. Active therapeutic social work through direct work with clients forms the major part of the third role of social work in community care set out above, and may also be an important aspect of the other two roles. It seems worthless to arrange for people to live in their own homes or in an attractive community setting rather than an oppressive institution, and then fail to help them make the best of their lives and skills. Equally, it seems pointless to arrange residential care, and not to provide a stimulating and worthwhile environment for those who use it. At every stage of looking at social work in community care, we need to examine the role of the counselling and therapeutic aspect of social work.

Counselling and therapeutic work are not, however, at the centre of the social work role as it is defined within present community care policy, even though counselling may be done, and all social work, including residential care, needs to be approached therapeutically. Although all social work activities have similar aims, many of them are concerned with making clients' lives happier or more efficient by indirect action, by affecting services and resources in the community. The Barclay Report (1982) called this 'social care planning', which bears a close relationship to the idea of 'community social work' (Hadley *et al.*, 1987).

For example, John is a young man who suffers from cerebral palsy.

Compared with most of us, his body is twisted, he makes unco-ordinated movements of his limbs, and his speech is indistinct and hard to follow for people who do not know him well. He would like to become more involved in social activities for his age group, and with the encouragement of a local priest, he attends a church youth club, but finds communication difficult, and is not involved in many of the informal activities which take place there, although he is accepted into formal events. One or two of the other members have told the priest that they find his presence frustrating and in-hibiting, although they have tried to be polite. The direct way of dealing with this might be to help John accept the limitations of his disabilities, find alternative, perhaps specialised, clubs where he will be more acceptable and offer social skills training and therapy aimed at improving his communication and ability to cope in general social situations.

But this is not enough, for two reasons. First, it makes no con-tribution to the resources of the community which will resolve other such problems in the future. The organisation of the club which permits such events, the attitudes of the other youngsters, the ob-trusiveness of disability in ordinary social settings and the capacity of the staff and members of the club to deal with these feelings and problems – none of these issues is dealt with. So similar difficulties could arise over some other disability next year, and the same rig-marole would have to be endured again. The second reason why the direct response is not enough is that it places most of the re-sponsibility for dealing with what has gone wrong upon John. He has to learn the skills and manage his feelings. People have to re-strict their range of responses in order to be loving and caring to him, and this may produce unreal relationships – they feel the need to be tolerant, and cannot criticise or deal with him naturally. This is unfair to him, and may lead to longer-term feelings of bitterness or distortion of attitudes and relationships. Backlash attitudes like this often get in the way of attempts to reduce prejudice and dis-crimination and respond in an anti-discriminatory way to stigma-tising disabilities. Responsibility and action should be taken by someone other than John to deal with the problem at its source.

Direct counselling work – however effective with clients may in this way individualise problems which have wider ramifications, and prevent us from doing work which helps a wider group of peo-ple with related problems. We also deal with problems which have multiple causes deriving from a variety of different people by working only with one person, treating the problem as individual, rather than accepting the extent of responsibility. Very often this leads us wrongly to see the individual as *the* problem. Indirect work through social care planning recognises the complexity of the problems and the extent of the social networks which are often involved in the creation and maintenance of problems. Acting in this way is an essential part of fulfilling the second role of social work in community care practice, that of developing community resources through community social work so that they are appropriate to the needs of actual and potential clients of community care services.

The first role of social work in community care policy, care management, links these two roles of social work – the individual 'counselling' aspect and the community-oriented 'social care planning' aspect of the Barclay Report. It is a way of organising the service which attempts to tie service planning and development with individual needs. It particularly relies on assessment skills which have traditionally formed an important basis of social work activities. While there is no assumption, in policy terms, that care management will always be done by social workers – there are different views about this – social workers' experience, breadth of awareness of service and their socially-oriented training suggests that social work skills are particularly relevant to care management. Their professional role in social services departments (SSDs), the lead public agency involved in implementing community care policy, will always make them a major contributor to care management where it is undertaken by multi-disciplinary teams or by people whose background is in other professional areas.

Complexity and multiple responsibility are not the only issues. Individual, direct work may be preferred to more broadly-based indirect work because of personal interest, but also because of power differentials. Many people who suffer the consequences of social and personal problems over a long period are and feel powerless. This is because they come to form part of groups in society which are devalued by many of the rest of us, because their physical or mental condition (such as physical or mental disorders), or their social situation (such as living on a much criticised housing estate), or their physical characteristics (such as coming from a minority ethnic community) have come to be more important to us than their individuality. We feel that difference from some conventional norm

represents someone of low value, and we use the power of the majority
to discriminate against and oppress those who are different. Therefore, in our preference for working with individuals we are falling
in with the social expectations which stigmatise and oppress people
in the groups that we deal with. We are part of a set of institutionalised assumptions which underlie such obvious manifestations of
oppression as racism and sexism.

This issue is important for community care practice because of
the client groups which are the objects of community care policy.
Direct counselling work is inadequate because community care particularly bears on oppressed groups in society, and so requires the
broader approach to social work which indirect work through social
care planning implies. To understand why this is, we need to understand what community care is about, and why it has developed as
the principal social care policy for these oppressed client groups.

Outlining policy: Chapters 1 and 2

The first two chapters of this book will explore community care
policy in two different ways. This chapter explores the broad out-
lines of community care policy and the various elements within it.
We shall be returning to many of these throughout the book. I identify a number of elements of community care policy and relate them
to the concept of 'community'. Then I explore some of the policy
issues which arise around each element. Finally, I analyse the social
work role and argue for the value of social worker's skills, knowledge
and training as the basis of an important role in community care.

Chapter 2 looks at the historical development of the policy and
maps out social work's place within that history. This leads to the
identification of three social objectives of present policy. We return
to these again, in the final chapter, which looks forward and asks
whether we can see these objectives being achieved by present policy.

The policy meaning of community care

'Community care' is a government policy, expressed in a White
Paper and extended policy guidance, and implemented through a
recent Act of Parliament (the *National Health Service and Com-*

munity Care Act, 1990 [*NHS&CCA*]). This requires services for certain client groups of the health and social services in Britain to be organised and provided in certain ways. The policy has the following main points.

- It covers people with long-term care needs.
- De-institutionalisation is an important aim. This means that people who have been living in and have been provided with caring services in large institutions are likely to be moved outside them. The overall number and size of such institutions should be reduced. People who might have entered institutions for care will be in institutions for briefer periods or will be cared for completely outside them.
- A 'mixed economy of care' will be created where public, voluntary or not-for-profit, informal and private providers of care interact with each other, exchanging potential clients and resources. This aspect of the policy reflects a characteristic approach to the management of state services taken by the Conservative governments of the 1980s and 1990s.
- Informal care has priority. As a result, there will be more and closer relationships between people who are cared for by social and health services and relatives, friends, neighbours, informal carers and volunteers outside institutions.
- It aims to increase citizen participation and choice in who provides caring services and how it is done.
- Services will be 'needs-led', so that care will be provided according to an assessment of the needs of the people concerned, rather than directing them towards a set and limited range of services.
- An important aim is to contain the rising costs of social care, while providing services to more people.

'Community' in community care policy

These aspects of community care policy reflect various conceptions of the nature of 'community'. Confusion about ideas of community has been an aspect of social and political debate since the nineteenth century. The following are important landmarks of this debate.

- Tönnies's (1955 – originally 1887) formulation of the ideas of 'community' (*gemeinschaft*) and 'association' (*gesellschaft*), the first implying closely integrated groups of people, the second fragmented and divided societies, with the implication that the former is preferable;
- a variety of studies of communities in the 1950s and 1960s using anthropological methods, many summarised in Klein (1965). These have led to the suggestion that some traditional communities which had been in existence a long time created a warmer and more integrated style of living, in which families and neighbours supported one another closely. Crow and Allan (1994) argue that these have been disproportionately influential in developing ideas of 'community';
- anxiety from the 1930s onwards that because of extensive changes in housing and other economic changes such as the decline of traditional industries, the quality of this supposed traditional community life was being damaged, and the development of planning mechanisms to control physical development of towns;
- cultural analysis, such as that of Williams (1983, pp. 75–6) which regarded 'community' (although originally implying 'the common people and shared relations') as a 'warmly persuasive word' with no countervailing opposite and which must therefore always be positive in its connotations;
- the concern of sociologists that as a result of the political, policy and social implications of the use of 'community' it could not be used as the basis for rigorous study of social life (see, for example, Stacey, 1969);
- attempts to respond to social pressures in inner cities by special projects to develop a mutually supportive community where it was presumed not to exist, and through 'community politics' focused on local issues. The most famous of these projects were the 'community development projects' of the 1970s.

Central to all these debates is the idea that there is or should or might be a form of living which feels warm and supportive to its participants. In this way of living, there is solidarity between people who share interests or aspects of their lives. Often this solidarity is supported by proximity: life is carried on in the same locality. Networks, the social links between people, are closely integrated, so that people in a community see and interact with each other a lot.

An important aspect of political debate about this concept of community is the assumption that it once existed in many places and has been lost to a greater or lesser extent.

These ideas have, of course, influenced social work and the social services. Social and political debate presumes that if community were present, there would be less need for social services, so the social objective of creating or recreating community has become part of many public services, including social work. Moreover, the 'warm, persuasive' terminology has been taken into social work and various therapies. We talk about 'therapeutic communities', for example, to refer to a particular way of organising residential and day care establishments and hospitals (Millard, 1992). Within social work and social policy, there are a number of distinctive meanings of 'community' to be aware of.

One meaning of 'community' distinguishes it from the state (meaning an expression through organised political structures of the will of the people) and the community as an expression of people's collective actions. In this distinction, 'community' implies ownership by the people involved rather than the separateness implied by provision through organised, politically-defined collective provision. Baldwin (1993) argues, for example, that a new model of care had grown up which rejects 'locality' as the basis for community in favour of the solidarity of relationships. He defines 'community' in his model of community care as residing in very local networks, with closely interacting relationships between multi-disciplinary teams and empowered service users. This model originates from a 'bottom-up' perspective, deriving from citizen and clients' rights action groups responding to 'top-down' government during the 1980s.

Related to this within community care and other community policies is a shift from collective provision, which is often associated with more socialist ideologies. There has been a move towards more personal responsibility which is often associated with 'New Right' ideologies which have been influential in the Conservative governments of the 1980s and 1990s. Mayo (1994) notes how changes towards a 'mixed economy' of welfare have implied different conceptualisations of 'community' and consequently of activities such as community work.

A further meaning is concerned with locality. One aspect of community care policy in the 1990s is that it intends to be locally rather than centrally planned and organised. On the other hand, unlike health service trusts and grant-maintained schools which are 'opted out' from, respectively, health authority and local authority control, community care will still be the subject of a local authority plan, with a wide range of services organised into a network of provision rather than simply a collection of independently managed units. Elements of localised responsiveness and localised authority for provision and policy are implied by applying the term 'community' to community care.

Another conception of 'community' is that of 'community of interest'. It is assumed that community care provides for groups of people with identifiable interests. Thus, 'de-institutionalisation' assumes that all groups of people who are being discharged from long-stay care institutions will have similar interests which justify providing a similarly organised service. Cutting across this interest group, it is assumed that identified groups of people such as elderly people, people with physical disabilities and people with mental illness or learning disabilities will each have shared interests which can be planned for coherently.

'Community' can also mean 'non-institutional' and informal rather than officially-organised care. These are distinctions noted by Bayley (1973) as meaning care *in* the community in smaller institutions but still by professional staff as opposed to care *by* the community outside institutions but by informal carers.

Finally, 'community' is used as a political and ideological term. Willmott (1989) has shown how it is frequently attached to services which have elements of local organisation to exact commitment from people by the feeling of involvement and connection that is offers. Although this sometimes gains approval for official services by emphasising their 'community' nature, it may also seek to emphasise the element of personal commitment and action expected of citizens. In this way, attaching 'community' to community care might signal to people that they should give approval of it as a concept, and might also press them (perhaps wrongly) to take personal greater responsibility in providing informal care than they would if another term were used.

The elements of community care policy

People of all political views would probably agree with my summary of the main points of community care policy, but controversy about the nature of 'community' raises many issues about the meaning of this policy to ordinary people. There are important sociological issues about the nature of community and responsibility to care in our society and how people understand 'community', 'need' and 'caring responsibilities'. It also raises political and philosophical issues about the role of 'formal' official care in relation to informal care, and this is inextricably bound up with changes in social expectations and the costs of implementing the policy. This becomes clear as soon as we look at each of the points made above concerning what the policy is about.

Long-term care

Community care policy is about people who need long-term care, but as it is generally understood and organised in SSDs there are complications. Most children and young people are excluded, because they are covered by different legislation (mainly, the *Children Act, 1989*), but some community care plans do include information about them. Government guidance emphasises the similarity in approach between the community care and children's legislation (DoH, 1990, para. 1.18). This view has been criticised. For example, Stace and Tunstill (1990) argue that the approach of the two pieces of legislation and their context is significantly different. Child care legislation derives from criminal justice, marital breakdown and child welfare laws; it is protective and limits choice for the client, who is clearly defined as the child. Community care legislation provides a much less comprehensive range of powers to provide welfare services for an indistinct client group. Policy debate in community care often confuses clients' needs and wishes with those of their carers. The care management approach and 'mixed economy of care' are not used in the children's legislation. Some categories of client overlap. Disabled children, for example, are usually regarded as coming more within community care than child care. Defining responsibilities may be a problem where parents receive community care services, where there are young carers (for example, children caring for a disabled parent) and where children (for example, those with learning difficulties) transfer to adult services when the special status of childhood ends.

   Hallett (1991) makes similar but different points. She argues that the *Children Act, 1989* is based on a wide professional consensus,

whereas the community care legislation reflects Conservative government views of the role of social care and the state within it. She also
notes that the children's reforms have developed complex and bureaucratic procedures in the public sector, while the community care legislation seeks to avoid this. However, the emphasis on user participation
is similar in both areas. I argue later that this is because the government seeks to use it to control mistrusted professional discretion.

Community care are being about long-term care does not cut it
off from all other forms of care. When does someone need 'long-
term' rather than 'short-term' or 'acute' care? For example, some
people who have a mental illness have periods when their condition
is active and vigorous medical treatment may be needed. This is
usually regarded as an 'acute' episode. However, if such episodes
recur, the overall mental condition of the patient may deteriorate,
and they become less able to manage a fairly normal life; so they
may come to need long-term care. One of the controversies of community care policy for many years has been concerned with how
such people may become 'revolving door' patients, constantly in
and out of hospital for treatment periods. Often, their overall capacity to manage their lives is never examined and supported. This
throws stress on them, their relatives, friends and neighbours and
fails to provide for long-term needs.

Also, not everyone needing long-term care is included in community care policy. Some people who need long-term hospital care
would not be considered as part of community care, because long-
term provision in a health care institution is not regarded as 'in the
community'. At the other end of the scale of needs, an elderly woman
who needs minimal weekly home help assistance is certainly being
provided with a social service, but it is doubtful whether she is
being provided with 'care'. In many areas she would not be included in community care.

There is also a political and policy issue about the distribution of
resources to long-term and acute care. If there are limited resources
and community care is about emphasising long-term care in competition with acute care, there is the possibility of a reduction in acute
services, or a reduction in the rate of increase in provision of acute
services. So emphasising community care may imply difficult decisions about the level of provision elsewhere. Certainly this has been
government policy for many years, even though it has not been
successfully achieved.

De-institutionalisation

Community care policy aims to remove care from institutions, and prevent people from being required to receive services from within buildings. It is concerned with de-institutionalisation not only from buildings, but also from ways of organising care which increase dependency in other ways. First, the policy prefers care to be provided outside institutions; that is, buildings whose main or only purposes are to offer care.

Second, if care is provided in buildings, its organisation should be relatively open and unrestrictive, so that its clients and workers can move backwards and forwards relatively easily, and their life-styles can be as uncontrolled by the building's environment as possible. This second aim seeks to move away from the evils of what Goffman (1961) calls 'total institutions' in which most aspects of living are catered for from within a single building-based institution.

Third, the whole service within which care is provided should be relatively open, flexible and unstructured, not arranged into a set pattern. This meaning of de-institutionalisation is concerned with the whole pattern of provision, rather than just its setting. One of the factors in flexible provision is the people who provide care and the methods that they use. Community care policy assumes that professionally-controlled methods and personnel will not be the main focus of provision, unless this is made necessary by the needs of the person concerned.

It is an extreme view which says that no institutional care should be provided at all. For people with extensive needs, care in a protected environment may be the most appropriate course. Moreover, institutions may provide 'asylum' to which people under pressure in ordinary life may escape to a more secure setting, whether for a short or long period (Murphy, 1991, p. 146). Institutions might be organised in more open or therapeutic ways. They can use a variety of staff skills and get patients involved to an extent that might be difficult in a community setting, where it is sometimes harder to bring extensive resources to bear. If people have become 'institutionalised', that is, so used to institutional living that they have lost the skills and motivation for independent living, they may need the continued support of institutional living. This may also be true for people whose disability, behaviour or intelligence means that they cannot manage independently. Some people may need protecting

from exploitation in ordinary life, or others might need protection
from their own behaviour or difficulties. However, as Bean and
Mounser (1993) point out, under community care policy, most patients
in mental hospitals, who might formerly have expected to stay there
for long periods, will be provided with care primarily in the community. They might be moved back into hospital if their needs become serious for an 'acute' episode.

The policy of de-institutionalisation can, therefore, be as controversial as that of long-term care. An important debate has centred
on the run-down and closure of mental hospitals in Britain and other
countries in Europe and the USA (Bean and Mounser, 1993; Brown,
P., 1985; Murphy, 1991; Ramon and Giannichedda, 1988; Tomlinson,
1991) and the effects of this, especially on people with long-term
mental illness. Although there is evidence that patients would prefer living independently, there has also been evidence that services
in the community have not been extensive enough to support people who have been discharged. Where they have returned to live
with parents and other relatives, sometimes the pressure of their
problems and behaviour has adversely affected their family's quality
of life.

One result of changes in hospital provision has been changes in
the rights accorded to people with mental illness. Tomlinson (1991)
bases his theoretical framework for understanding the 'retreat from
the asylum' on changes in the nature of authority in the management of services, from a more centralised system towards decentralised services, and eventually, it might be hoped, services where
consumers have a higher degree of choice and control. However,
Bean and Mounser (1993) argue that, while the 'right to treatment'
implied in the availability of mental hospitals often reflected authoritarian and medical conceptions of treatment in which patients
had little say, more decentralised 'community' options may remove
the certainty that help will be provided at all. Barham (1992, p. 137)
places at the centre of his analysis of 'closing the asylum' changing
perceptions of mental patients from a position of seeing them as
disabled, needing caring by professionals who are 'part of the system' towards a position in which they are seen as citizens in a diverse range of services, where professionals 'struggle to develop
autonomy for users'. Phil Brown (1985, pp. 204–5) argues that greater
concern for patients' rights derives from political and economic
pressures to reduce costs (leading to an emphasis on patients' inde-

pendence), and professionals' concentration on humanitarianism to justify demands for financial support for improving treatments programmes. Institutional reform, in his view, derives from the need to develop clear treatment goals for patients. The philosophy of 'normalisation' (Ramon, 1988, 1991; Towell, 1988; Brown and Smith, 1992) is one change in professional thinking which seeks to develop greater opportunities for patients' rights and participation within a non-institutional approach (see, particularly, Chapter 7 below).

Another debate is concerned with the restricted life which may be led by people who are discharged from long-term care, or are unable to get support from a comprehensive range of services in the community. In a large institution, people with mental illnesses or with learning disabilities may have an extensive social life, with good leisure facilities and immediately available support. They are relatively free from exploitation by ill-intentioned or inconsiderate members of the public. When they are discharged to live in the community, they are usually on social security benefits and are living in small-scale developments, often group homes of three or four people. They therefore do not have enough money to follow a very active life, and take advantage of general leisure provision, which is usually commercially run and priced for those who are able to work. They are also cut off from contact with larger numbers of people from their own backgrounds, and may be exploited or stigmatised by neighbours or people in the local public house.

Much the same points might be made of people who have never been in long-term institutional care. An elderly or disabled person may lose contact with friends and family, have very little opportunity to make social contacts among people who share their problems, and may be irritating to and out of touch with younger or physically able people who live around them. They and others around them might prefer institutional care.

Community care policy aims at de-institutionalisation from health service institutions because these have a history of being most expensive and most dependency-creating in their inmates. However, health service institutions are not necessarily so. There has also been a debate about what kinds of living arrangement consitute de-institutionalisation. When we talk we talk about 'institutions' we tend to think of Victorian buildings with echoing halls, high-ceilinged wards and rows of closely-packed beds. We are less disapproving of more modern hospitals where facilities fit modern treatment

assumptions more readily, but they may be equally oppressive or
disorientating to many patients. Short-stay institutions are more acceptable because they do not create the level of dependence implied by long-stay regimes. Some health authorities, though, have
sought to set up smaller more human-scale units for caring for long-
stay patients. There are treatment methods, such as therapeutic communities (Blood, *et al.*, 1988; Clark, 1964; Jansen, 1980; Jones, M.,
1968; Kennard, 1983; Righton, 1979) which seek to make use of
the nature of an institution and the fact of being in it as part of a
treatment process designed to improve human functioning both within
the institution and in moving towards life outside it. On the other
hand, there are modern, human-scale institutions run by local authorities where routines reflect the staff's convenience rather than the
residents' needs for flexible care. These complexities lead Baldwin
et al. (1993) to argue that the idea of institutionalisation has out-
lived its usefulness, and that a range of settings needs to be explored, in relation to the extent to which they create dependency,
independence and interdependence. This takes us on to the next aspect
of community care policy.

Reducing dependence on public care

This element of community care policy contains two aspects: dependence and public care.

We have seen that one of the arguments for de-institutionalisation is that care in institutions makes residents less capable of managing their own lives both within the institutions and, if they get
the opportunity, outside it. Most care in institutions is public care,
either because it is directly provided by public bodies such as health
or social services authorities, or because much of it has been paid
for from the public purse, for example, by social security allowances, replaced in the new policy by payments from SSDs. If people are made unnecessarily dependent they make equally unnecessary
demands on the public purse.

This is not all. Conservative ideology would suggest that having
services which induce dependence on public provision has undesirable effects in the wider population and social institutions. It tends
to lead to an acceptance that it is the state's responsibility to provide for people in difficulties, rather than inducing people to work
harder to get out of difficulties themselves, or encouraging people

to help their relatives and friends without invoking the state. In turn, extensive public services create occupational groups with an interest in maintaining and increasing their power and influence by extending the services they provide; in turn this induces more dependence. Eventually, these developments lead to the state having to make increasing provision, burdening tax expenditure to the point where the economy cannot support it.

Although community care policy is not a direct implementation of such a philosophy, since it has been built up over many decades and contains many different strands of thought, it has developed strongly in the 1980s and 1990s while a government has been in power which has sympathy with such views. That philosophy is reflected in the strength of effort put behind its implementation and aspects of it which encourage the development of a 'mixed economy of care' with a strong role for the private sector, and a withdrawal of direct provision by public authorities. An example of the sort of response which results was the withdrawal of the generously funded Independent Living Fund, and the replacement of it, in 1993, for people not already receiving grants with much more restricted provision (DoH/DSS, 1993). As a result, expenditure was reduced, and service provision was worsened for an important group of service users who are often discriminated against in ordinary social life and in arrangements for public services.

A crucial element of reducing dependence on public care is the consequences for the rights of citizens to collective provision for their welfare through state provision. Community care policy, in that it promotes informal care, voluntary and private sector involvement in care and possibly fragmented systems of provision can be seen as a part of a movement to focus on individualised rights of citizens, rather than collective rights. This issue is explored in Chapter 2, as part of the argument that modern community care policy is individualising rather than collective in character; in Chapters 5 and 6 in relation to the development of informal, volunteer and independent sector provision; and in Chapter 8 on accountability and effectiveness. It is thus a theme which runs through the discussion of community care policy and practice in this book.

The Conservative government's ideology does not only affect the nature of services provided but also leads to a distinctive 'management approach'. This may involve 'privatisation', meaning that some formerly public services are sold to private (that is, for-profit) operators, or private operators may be induced to become part of systems of care which were previously wholly public. More commonly in the social services, which are not very amenable to private provision, the government's management approach has led to 'marketisation'. In this process, elements of a public system are costed and established as separate units which can complete against one another, or buy (either notionally or actually) services from one another. This is said to encourage efforts by public service providers to consider and drive down the costs of what they offer, and to improve the quality of it. In many different services, a process of 'compulsory competitive tendering', 'market-testing', budgetary devolution and 'purchaser-provider splits' in the organisation of services are signs of this approach. In some cases, such as the local management of schools, it is allied with local devolution which encourages more 'community involvement' to restrain professional control of services – in this example, teachers' control being restrained by parents. Robyn Lawson (1993) identifies the three key areas of change for social services management as a result of government management policies as:

● measures to match services to needs;
● measures to promote choice, flexibility and innovation; and
● measures to promote value for money, efficiency, accountability and quality.

Informal care

Public, private and voluntary sectors are not the only parts of the 'mixed economy of care'. Community care policy seeks to encourage 'informal' care by friends, neighbours and relatives of people in need of care. There are a number of reasons for this (which are explored further in Chapter 5).

● The *carers revolution* of the 1980s (see, for example, Richardson *et al.*, 1989; House of Commons Social Services Committee, 1990) led to the recognition that most care is informal, and that stressful demands on these carers had been neglected by public social services, which did not connect well with and support their efforts. There is a power element to the neglect of informal carers. Many of them are women, and there are gender stereotypes that place a moral and social responsibility on them to provide care within the family and neighbourhood, and their needs in fulfilling such responsibilities were not well-recognised by powerful, patriarchal institutions in the public social services.

● Professional care is *expensive* where informal arrangements have collapsed or are insufficient. Some expenditure on supporting informal care is therefore justified on economic grounds.

● Informal care is *flexible*. Carers often live in the same house or neighbourhood as the person in need and can respond as and when required, whereas visiting professionals can only be available according to pre-existing schedules or in emergencies.

● Informal care is very often *preferred* by people in need because there are long-standing relationships and exchanges between them and their carers which has built up a feeling of mutual responsibility. However, this is not always so. There is a potential conflict of interest between carers and those who are cared for. While things go well, an informal care arrangement may be the best option. But where people feel forced to care by social expectations or because there are no alternatives and no support, it may be unpleasant for the carer and this may disadvantage the person cared for. One consequence may be physical or other abuse of the person being cared for. There have also been examples of exploitation of elderly or disabled people for financial gain. There is a lot of evidence of older people feeling forced into residential care because of family pressures. It cannot be assumed that the felt obligation to care will always be accepted by informal carers, or that caring responsibilities are accepted altruistically or by choice. Very often, the arrangement to care will be a social bargain, with the inconvenience for the carers set against past social obligations between them and the person being cared for or the relief of social or family pressures which makes a carer feel they must care even if they do not wish to do so.

Underlying all these reasons for enchancing informal care is, again, a political and ideological assumption. Henwood and Wicks (1985) argue that differences in view about whether community care should lead to more strongly-developed social planning for care or less intervention by the state through marketisation come down to a fundamental difference in view about the nature of 'family' and its role in society. Right-wing ideology seeks to present the 'family'

and 'neighbourhood' essential parts of the fabric of society, which
help to cement social relationships and maintain social order and
conventional social relationships. Encouraging the acceptance of
social obligations which come from family and community relationships of this kind is seen in this view to support society and to be
a moral and social 'duty'. Such a view assumes an existing order in
which those without economic power to buy care and those, such
as women, who are socially expected to provide care must comply
with such conventional social assumptions. A more radical view (for
example, Dalley, 1988) would see caring as a collective responsibility in which the state would take on the obligation for supporting
family and informal care, in order to fulfil that collective responsibility. This view would accept state provision as an appropriate choice
for care provision, rather than as a last resort in the event of the
failure of informal care.

Increased participation and choice

One of the aims of community care policy is to promote the opportunity of the people involved to make their choices. This policy
comes from a number of sources.

One is a developing professional ideology. Social work has always
had a commitment to values such as 'self-determination' of clients,
but recently there has been a wider acceptance of clients' rights to
participation in social work process and decisions which has sometimes been incorporated into legislation and official guidance. This
is strongly so in the case of community care policy.

Another source of the movement towards participation is a developing consumer movement, taken up in some ways by Conservative
ideology. More widely in society, a consumer movement has developed which is concerned to protect consumers of goods and services from exploitation by providers who have excessive power in
relation to consumers (Kroll and Stampfl, 1981, p. 97). However,
there are major differences in public sector provision. Generally,
the consumer's problem in the public sector is that the provider has
to ration services and may damage the consumer's interests in unfair rationing. In commercial life the provider has exactly opposite
aims: to sell as much as possible. Here, the consumer needs help in
making choices and protection from exploitation by unfair or unsafe selling and manufacturing methods. Protection is still relevant

in the public sector, but much participation is concerned with providing a brake on professional or bureaucratic behaviour.

A third source of the movement towards participation is evidence of the failure among professionals to consider the wishes of people being cared for and their carers.

The government's objective of a mixed economy of care raises questions about the policy of choice, however. 'Choice' in this context derives from a market view which says that competition among services must lead to their improvement, because they will improve provision and reduce price in order to remain 'in business'. This will only be so if there are enough services to choose from. Where the total service is inadequate, people or purchasers of service have to pay inflated prices or choose services which do not met their needs because that is all that is available. Most private services are in residential care, for example, so that competition in home care may not be available. The government, recognising this, has had to encourage the independent residential care sector to diversify into domiciliary care (KPMG Peat Marwick, 1993) and direct local authorities to include arrangements for purchasing non-residential care from the independent sector in their community care plans (see Chapter 8 below and DoH, 1994a). Also, most choice will be available to those with more money, and if there is poor financing of a scheme whereby public money buys care on behalf of those who do not have enough resources of their own, publicly-financed service users may get an inadequate service simply because of that. Although it is not unreasonable that those with money should be able to buy *additions* to service, many people think that choice of a *satisfactory* service should not be restricted to those who can pay.

Finally, the development of advocacy, and particularly ideas of self-advocacy – where service users come together to support each other in advocating for their needs within service development and as individuals – which are associated with professional movements such as normalisation (both as a fundamental value and method in social work and as a need for community care clients) has strengthened the movement for participation. This is explored more fully in Chapter 7.

Needs-led services

The policy that community care services should be needs-led comes
from two major sources:

- the assumption that previously local authorities through their social
  workers tended to assess new clients for services that were available, rather than services which might be, but were not, made
  available or which were not available but might be needed by
  the client;
- the concern that where social security allowances towards the
  cost of fees for residential care in the private sector were available, people might choose to take up this provision and the allowance, when, had they been assessed for local authority care,
  they would not have been regarded as being 'in need' of the
  service.

This second source of the needs-led policy draws attention to the
essentially contested and political nature of decisions about needs.
Once something is defined as a 'need', rather than, say, a 'want'
we tend to feel an emotional pressure to meet it. This means that
defining something as a 'need' makes it seem more necessary than
before to take action to deal with it; so a 'need' seems to require
the allocation of resources more strongly than something which is
not. Assessing need thus becomes associated with political pressure
to provide services, and with rationing services.

   Bradshaw (1972) developed a taxonomy of need, which sets out
different sorts of need which would have different consequences for
how we would provide services:

- *normative need,* defined by the expert or professional;
- *felt need,* which is the same as a client's wants;
- *expressed need,* where felt need is turned by an action, such as
  applying for services, into demand;
- *comparative need,* where people are assumed to be in need if
  they suffer the same conditions as others do who receive a service.

Clayton (1983) criticises this taxonomy on practical and other grounds,
arguing that it cannot help us turn a better understanding of need
into decisions about whether or not to supply a service. Gilbert Smith

(1980) showed in a study of a social services department that need is constructed administratively by the decisions of social workers as they go about their daily business. Kemshall (1986) studied an intake team in a social services office and showed that decisions about need were constructed by workers' everyday reactions to the problems that they faced, by reinterpreting the official definitions of needs that their department gave them according to a social consensus among themselves.

The uncertainty about what need is suggests that as soon as we move from 'felt need' we enter a political world in which decisions are actually conditioned by resources, and this makes the cost implications of community care policy a crucial issue to consider.

Costs

Much debate about community care centres around the costs of long-term care services. I reduced all the complexity of this issue above to a statement that community care policy sought to 'contain' costs while providing for more people. We need to disentangle a number of points. The easiest way to do this is to start from 'institutions', since community care is a policy of moving away from institutions as a form of social care provision.

Institutions are generally cheaper than community provision because clients and care providers can be grouped together for specialised care, thus cutting down the time and cost (to the service, not the client or their visitors) of travel to receive a service. The Victorian history of using institutions as a deterrent to induce 'good behaviour' among the working class reduces demand for services through stigma. Once institutions are built, the continuing cost of providing services within them is quite cheap and inflation reduces the real cost of the loans which paid the capital cost of building them.

However, these advantages are not absolute or continuing. Older institutions become more unsuitable over time for modern patterns of care and of living, and are expensive to upgrade and maintain. Once there, they have to be maintained, and this sucks money out of the care system, meaning that others with lesser needs can have fewer resources. If institutions are the centre of provision, they therefore attract more clients who do not need expensive, specialised care and who would be more cheaply provided for with a mixture of informal care and minimal professional support. These people may grow dependent on the institutional care, and so become more costly than if they and their carers were funded to maintain independence. The numbers of people needing care are increasing, because of population changes and improvements in treatment (see Chapters 2 and 5), so the demands on and costs of institutions are multiplied and the potential saving of a more differentiated system of care will grow.

We can now see the financial justification for community care. Rising costs of institutions, better treatment and professional and personal preferences lead to pressure to move people from institutions and prevent admission to them. This leads to a larger number of people in the community needing care, which is only cheaper if the amount of care is reduced below the crossover point where it becomes cheaper to deal with them *en masse* in an institution. However, more care is difficult to provide within a constrained budget because of the costs of existing institutions. A rising population in need of care thus increases the cost justification for community care, because although the overall need for care in the population must rise, since there are more people in the categories of those who tend to need care, keeping them out of institutions and helping them remain independent (even at some cost) will reduce the speed with which costs rise. If by doing this we reduce the overall need for institutions, more substantial savings may be possible, by closing some of the institutions and selling the buildings or the land on which they are built. This can pay for some of the costs of the services which have allowed the institution to close.

Overall costs rather than part of the picture must be considered. For example, if the health service closes an institution, it saves money. If the people who leave or can no longer enter it need more social services or social security allowances, these services cost more. As costing has become more sophisticated, some of these counterbalancing costs have been identified, so that a more complicated picture of the real cost advantages can be built up. Netten and Smart (1993) have produced detailed unit costs for a wide variety of services which compare costs per day or per week. These show that generally hospitals are more expensive than nursing homes, which in turn cost more than residential care. Day and home care may be more interchangeable. These figures for 1992 are part of an annual publication which will be a useful resource in evaluating the costs of their provision.

Even so, non-financial costs are often unconsidered. Examples might be distress or pressure on people in need or their informal carers, who *can* cope, but suffer more if they have to. Also, financial costs may be borne by non-relevant services (such as transport or education) which may have to cope with more difficult people, and by clients and their carers themselves. Another point is that even when small-scale provision increases costs, the quality of service and 'domestic' scale of life-style is more satisfactory to the people involved. However, it may be that the quality of what staff do is more important in all settings than the nature of the setting. Felce (1993) argues, in relation to residential care settings for people with severe learning disabilities, that even in an attractive 'ordinary housing' setting, staff inputs may not lead to effective outcomes for service users. In research in a similar setting, Mansell and Beasley (1993) show that keeping up quality of service and staff commitment is a difficult task.

There is evidence that, during the 1980s, increases in health care budgets in the UK have been insufficient to keep up with increases in need (Ham *et al.*, 1990). This raises the suspicion that all arguments about the advantages of community care may be subsidiary to the cost savings which may be inherent in its implementation. Against such a suspicion, it may be said that it is widely recognised that public preference for a non-institutionalised, good-quality community service is such that, if it were available, demand would rise so much that overall costs would continue to spiral upwards, in spite of the cost savings in relation to individual cases.

It is clear that the government hopes to use community care policy to prevent the rise in costs and provide for the rising demand for care in ways which will restrict increases in costs, thus dealing with more people for the same amount of money. This will throw greater burdens on informal carers, and perhaps some professionals, which will not be well accounted for in money terms. The policy may lead to reductions in provision which is socially valued (for example, hospital care, high-quality residential care) as the government withdraws money to use elsewhere. There may well be increases in provision (for example, home helps, day care) which is less well understood or which in some cases will not fully compensate for the apparent loss of service which might have provided more intensive care for those that needed it. On the other hand, such care might have been more heavily rationed, and the new provision offers some care to more people. Some groups in need of care (for example, people with mental illnesses) may be disadvantaged by being part of an undifferentiated service for more numerous groups (for example, elderly people). At the other end of the scale, concentrating services on deinstitutionalisation may remove valued resources from low-level provision, such as occasional home help for cleaning.

My overall judgement would be that the government hopes to provide more, better-quality services through implementing its community care reforms. It aims to reduce unnecessary costs in the system, particularly by reducing costs associated with unnecessary institutionalisation. Marketisation and care management will restrain inevitable increases in overall costs, by controlling demand. If this judgement is correct, the social work practice innovation of care management will constitute a major plank of the successful implementation of the government's policy and financial objectives. As well as this, *how* care management is implemented is crucial to the success of professional objectives in making the system more flexible and responsive to users' needs. It is crucial, in understanding community care policy, therefore, to explore the practice which will result and the role of social work within community care.

Social work skills in community care

This section draws together this discussion of the content of community care policy with the three social work roles in community care identified above. This enables us to discuss what social work offers to community care by identifying the particular social work skills which are relevant to this policy framework.

Table 1.1 sets out a useful way of understanding the elements of community care social work practice, starting from various types of social care that may be offered. The starting focus is on developing resources in the lives of clients. The second column identifies a range of resources that social workers might be working with. Each of these implies a type of social care practice, in column 1, associated with types of social work activity, and the extent of workers' involvement in the lives and environments of their clients. Each of these implies a continuum of activities. Practice might theoretically be activated from either end of the continua, or move outwards from

Table 1.1 *Types of social care and their role in community care*

Type of social care	Type of resources being used	Nature of social work activity	Range of workers' involvement	Position in community care practice
best use of client's resources	strengthening clients' own resources	enabling, support, protection	needs and environment of client	especially assessment and care planning
reducing conflict and uncertainty	family and informal network	negotiation, mediation	immediate family and social environment	especially care planning
finding and using resources effectively	organised services	creating, mobilising, linking resources	local network of services	plan implementation
promoting clients' interests	service management and planning	advocacy, empowerment	policy, management of services	care management, service planning and training
promoting political, social and service context	use and development of resources in society	promoting social action	broader social concerns	policy, service development

SOURCE: Payne, 1986a, pp. 3–5.

the middle. It is possible to look at the community and social context of care in a particular area, by understanding the range of services, the availability of informal care and then looking at the client's needs and wishes. However, we have seen that one of the crucial elements of community care policy is that it is needs-led and is concerned with helping clients and their carers to participate. The logic of this is that we must start any analysis from the client, and so the table places individual clients and their resources first, while not negating the alternative approach, which is the basis of community care planning for the range of services discussed in Chapter 9. In the last column, each level of activity is set against one of the commonly defined aspects of care management, so that the role of each type of activity at different stages of community care practice is identified, and readers can turn to relevant chapters in this book to see how community care policy seeks to implement social care activities and social work skills to improve clients' resources in that stage of community care.

Community care policy, then, sets a hierarchy of priorities, which I refer to as the 'community care tariff', discussed more fully in Chapter 5 (see Figure 5.1). It is preferred that the clients provide for themselves independently. If this is not possible, care ought, according to the policy, to be provided by informal carers or, lastly, through organised care. These are the elements that must be included in community care practice.

Before we can use skills for work with clients, we must understand the policy and service context of what we are trying to do. In this book, the policy context is covered by this chapter, which explores the content of community care policy and the role of social work within it, and by Chapter 2, which examines the development of community care policy and its links with social work. Understanding the crucial practice innovation of 'care management', covered in Chapter 3, is also an essential prerequisite, and policy contexts are included in later chapters concerned with practice developments, in particular the participation of service users and their carers in decision-making about the services and their own circumstances, which is relevant throughout, but particularly in Chapter 7. The organisational requirements for implementing community care policy are the major focus of Chapters 8 and 9. A crucial feature of these is the developing management techniques concerned with quality management. Although these are not directly associated with social work, they are having an increasing influence on management and particularly monitoring and review processes within social work.

Why should social workers be any more suitable than others to undertake many of these roles in the community care system? Fisher argues in relation to providing for dementia sufferers (1990a) and to working with carers (1990b) that effective use of social work skills is essential to making community care work well. In the same way, Biggs (1991) argues for the value of a personal and interactional psychodynamic approach to care management. This would, he argues, balance the tendency for care management to move away from a focus on face-to-face work with distressed people, its assumption that competing interests among the professionals are unproblematic, its assumption that there is a technical end-point of intervention in the delivery of a package of services and its emphasis on purchaser–

provider relationships rather than interpersonal relationships between worker and client.

The arguments for the value of social work fall into eight points:

- *The agency they are in* Social workers are the major professional group in social services departments, which have been identified as the lead agencies in implementing community care policy. The social work value system and skills are central to these agencies; the policy therefore values aspects of those values and skills. The relevant values which seem to align are the individualistic approach of social work (as opposed to a bureaucratic criteria-based process of decision-making) and the value base of creating independence among clients (rather than simply 'delivering' care).

- *The social model of practice* Social workers are educated primarily in the social and psychological sciences and focus on clients' social interactions in normal life, rather than having a medical or disease model directed towards 'curing' identified illnesses, which tends to be more common in the health and social care services. The social work approach is thus more appropriate to a policy of promoting independence and ordinary life than an approach which is more concerned with curing people who may be dependent because of illness or psychological problems.

- *Level of education* Social workers are educated at higher education level in a fairly wide range of relevant social sciences, rather than in a limited number of practical skills (as tends to be the case with lower-level care staff in social services) or in a particular service context (as with, say, nursing or housing staff), so they tend to have a wider awareness of services and social issues and be able to take in a broader range of issues than staff trained in other ways. This means that social workers are likely to be particularly flexible in implementing a policy which relies on taking a wide range of social factors and services into account.

- *Breadth of education and focus of practice* As a result of the breadth of their education and because of their role in public services generally, social workers tend to have training and experience in linking services and helping clients make use of the available services, rather than just providing their own professional skills. This fits well with the aims of community care policy.

- *Skills focus* Social work skills tend to be focused on inter-personal relationships and linking skills, rather than providing particular technical services or meeting caring needs. Social workers'skills thus seem especially relevant to a community care policy concerned with integrating a wide variety of services in a package for individual clients.

- *Assessment skills* Social work has been very widely used to assess complex social and psychological situations, in providing pre-sentence reports within criminal justice systems or social histories in psychiatric and a variety of other services. Assessment skills of this kind are crucial to the needs-led approach of community care. Unlike the assessment skills of some other professional groups, such as psychologists, social workers are trained with a social and interpersonal perspective, rather than a purely individualistic one. This again is particularly relevant to community care.

- *Risk orientation* Social work, partly because of its value system which aims at reducing dependence, tends to have more of an orientation to allowing clients to accept risks and follow their own path, rather than the caring, protective approach of many services with more of a medical model.

- *Participation orientation* Social work among caring occupations has more of a history of promoting participation by and advocacy for services users; this is probably because of the social science base of its training which tends to be more radical in focus than the medical or individualistic psychological model of many professionals in the health and social care fields.

I would not argue that social workers will always be the best people among a particular group of professional staff to undertake community care work. Particular activities and skills may be better implemented by another person in a particular case. I do argue that in general social work skills will offer more flexibility and breadth and a more appropriate approach than generally will be offered by any other professional group and by lower-level staff trained in particular skills.

Such a view is further borne out by the history of the development of community care, which, as we shall see in Chapter 2, is closely entwined with the history of the development of social work.

2

The Development of Community Care in the Social Services

Any understanding of the policy context of community care work must be, partly, historical. The pattern of a new service always derives from what has gone before, and the thinking which creates an innovation is a reaction against aspects of past provision, and must embrace favoured or necessary elements of former arrangements. Moreover, it must fit with other services which have not necessarily been changed and reflect political or management ideologies of the time. To act, we must know why we are here: this may cause us to rebel or seek to reconstruct what we do, or to acquiesce in or advance the flow of events.

Community care did not come to contain the elements discussed in Chapter 1 by coincidence or by intellectual innovation. It has been a long-standing part of social policy, and is a reaction to the trends of even longer ago. I argue in this chapter that community care came about partly as a reaction against institutional care. This is important for practice, because, by adopting community care as the focus of our policy and practice, we may overlook the value that institutional care needs to have in the provision of care services and fail to include it appropriately in our plans.

I also argue that the recent development of community care has been primarily concerned with the management and effective use of resources. This is important for practice, because it may cause the community care system to neglect the value of interpersonal relationships in making care services really effective and in supporting the commitment of informal carers.

In this chapter, four phases in the development of community care policy are identified, followed by an account of the issues which led to new policies being established during the 1980s. The fundamental argument, which is reviewed at the end of this account, is that policy developments of the 1980s represent a move away from commitment to community and collective responses to social need towards individualisation. Three historic aspects of community care policy and the role of social work within it are considered towards the end of the chapter.

Phases in the development of community care policy

Community care as a formal policy has been widely accepted in the UK since at least the 1950s. Its origins lie further back in the development of health and social services in the twentieth century. Parallels exist with policies for deinstitutionalisation in many other countries. It is not a policy without controversy, in spite of its wide acceptance among political parties and many professional ideologies.

The future implementation of community care policy has become intimately bound up with the future of the social and health services in Britain. This is because government decisions in this policy area tend to set out the role of the social services in relation to the health services, and also the relationship between the state social services, which have been the major providers of most types of social service, and the private and independent sectors, which have rapidly expanded in the field of residential care. This is likely to provide the launching pad for a greater emphasis on private and independent sector provision in social care. Their growth has shown that private sector provision of a major area of social service provision is possible, that there are people who will undertake it, and it has made an entirely new pattern of relationship between state and private sectors possible.

Table 2.1 sets out four phases which are useful for understanding the historical development of community care policy in the UK. This formulation emphasises, first, the central importance of institutions as the Victorian, post-Industrial Revolution response to social need. Reaction to this led to a growing emphasis on the idea of 'community' as the basis for a response to social need, and as a

Table 2.1 *Phases in the development of community care policy*

Period	Phase	Comment
To the end of the 19th century	*Institutional*	Main response to social need is to 'incarcerate' people in institutions
First part of 20th century	*Commitment*	Increasingly committed development of community response to social need
1960s and 1970s	*Community/ Collective*	Ideological commitment to 'community' in response to social need
1980s and 1990s	*Individual*	Shift from 'community' to emphasis on responding to individualised definitions of need

central concept from the 1950s onwards. Although 'community' is still important, from the 1980s policy has increasingly emphasised effective response to individual needs as the priority, although still within a non-institutional context. It is this emphasis on individualisation which supplies the political ideology behind increasing private and independent sector involvement in providing social care. Professional social work ideologies which maintain 'individualisation' of the needs of social work clients as an important value, rather than mutual and collective provision, tend to support the political ideology of individualism.

The institutional phase

The development of community care policy is a reaction to the use of institutions as an instrument of social policy. The first phase of response to social problems which began to develop during the Industrial Revolution in the UK and elsewhere was to set up institutions. They were to care for and control people when the breakdown of rural family and community life meant that care and the maintenance of social order from neighbours, friends and relatives was less available, particularly in the new industrial cities. Some services were needed simply because of awareness of a growing and unmanageable problem. The growth of lunatic asylums (the mental hospitals) and colonies (mental handicap hospitals for people with learning disabilities) is an example. The major institutions concerned were, however, the workhouses of the new Poor Law introduced in 1834.

These developments took place in a context, however, where it was assumed that the normal way of getting the necessities for maintaining life and health was through employment regulated by the economic market. Attempts were made to provide care through locally managed systems of support, within the old Poor Law in which local parishes took responsibility for income support and care of those without families to help them, but these failed. Failure came about because of increasing cost when the size of the problem increased, and because dependence on state help was fostered rather than employment in the market. An important aspect of the institutional system was, therefore, to affect the beliefs and regulate the attitudes and behaviour of the working class generally in order to avoid these problems (Parker, R., 1988).

So institutions were set up both to provide care and deal with growing social problems but also to control and reinforce a system of belief in the market and in the avoidance of dependence within the wider population. Institutional care has thus become associated with 'badness' and with dependence. One aspect of social work's professional origins lies in the staff of the workhouses. Many of the first employees of local authority welfare and children's departments after the Second World War started their careers under the Poor Law. The early almoners, who became medical social workers, grew out of a need to consider the social needs of patients in the hospitals of the late nineteenth and early twentieth centuries.

The commitment phase

The second phase of policy development was a long period of growing commitment to the idea of 'community' as the place for, and in some ways the instrument of, response to social needs, not as yet fully expressed in planned policy.

There was already a move away from institutions in ideas. Several child care agencies and some Poor Law institutions were using boarding out, where children were placed with individual families for care rather than being kept in homes (Packman, 1981). Between the wars, while the system remained much the same, legislation in the mental health field set the scene for treatment outside the asylums and colonies, though this was still not widespread. Psychiatric social work developed from the movement in the 1920s to provide alternative services in the community and for the asylums to become more outward-looking.

The major development in community care policy came in the welfare reforms following the Second World War. These established a social security system which was not based primarily on institutions, and the national health service. In the social services field, a welfare service for elderly and physically handicapped people included both field social work and residential care. These welfare services developed alongside a local authority social work service for children, with a policy of 'boarding out' children with foster parents rather than using residential care.

Developments in training for the children's departments, transplanted by the Younghusband Reports into training provision for workers in the welfare services, strengthened the role and standing of professional social work in local authority welfare services. This provided, in turn, the foundation for a movement to create a broad social work service within local government, which came to fruition in the implementation of the Seebohm Report (1968) and the establishment of local authority SSDs.

The 1950s also saw controversy about the role of institutions in the provision of long-term care in several fields. Theoretical and treatment developments, such as therapeutic communities, now made it possible to see institutions as having the capacity to be non-custodial, as therapeutic and as being beneficial to their inmates. It also made possible a confidence in non-medical forms of treatment outside hospital. Controversy about the poor standards of institutionalised care for elderly people arose following publication of Peter Townsend's 'The Last Refuge' (1962) and various scandals about institutional care occurred especially in the long-stay mental illness and mental handicap hospitals. The old buildings of the late nineteenth century were ending their useful life and becoming expensive to run.

Distaste for the dehumanising and unpleasant environments offered by the hospitals also evolved. Theoretical work by Goffman (1961) on total institutions (that is, those where all or most aspects of life were provided for within the institution) and Barton (1959) on the adverse effects of institutions on their inmates leading to what was described as 'institutional neurosis' was an important factor in the strengthening of these ideas.

The crucial series of events arose from the Percy Commission

(Percy Report, 1957) which examined the mental health services, coined the term 'community care' and proposed a new social work service for mentally ill and handicapped people, to be provided by local councils. The aim was to avoid unnecessary incarceration in mental hospitals by offering alternative services outside, and to provide after-care when patients were discharged.

These ideas were enacted in the *Mental Health Act, 1959*. As a result, the population in long-stay mental hospitals, already decreasing, continued to drop, and the concept of community care became associated particularly with the deinstitutionalisation of patients in mental hospitals.

The reasons for these changes in practice are controversial. Goodwin (1989) argues that they are not the result of improvements in drug treatment, which only served to maintain (and make possible its extension to more disturbed patients) an already existing run-down in hospital care, fuelled partly by the professional and ideological trends already noted. Neither was it a policy 'on the cheap' since, acording to Goodwin, costs have increased greatly as commitment to non-institutional services has grown. Goodwin argues that community care policy grew as a response to professional and political ideas, and because it enabled more patients to be treated (albeit more briefly) in a situation where awareness and understanding of mental illness was leading to an increase in patients needing treatment. In particular, he argues (Goodwin, 1990, p. 123) that government could not solve through institutional provisions the incompatibility between the need to control behaviour, to be seen as 'caring', and to legitimise the role of the state and the need to control costs.

In the health service, awareness of the never-ending demand for health services grew in the 1950s. The first attempts at planning came about and there was a considerable political impetus towards more rational use of resources and against poor quality care which was increasingly evident in the large hospitals. These led eventually to the health service reorganisation of the 1970s and 1980s. The post-war period also saw a development in caring services provided outside hospitals by the local authority health and welfare services set up after the end of the Poor Law. In the *Health Services and Public Health Act, 1968*, providing home help services was finally made a statutory duty for local authorities, recognising the *de facto* position.

The community phase

All these moves demonstrate the final stages of the shift from a fundamentally institutionally-based set of provisions to one which is commited to a community orientation. This constitutes the third phase of community care policy development. It is based on the philosophy of a 'community-collective' service. It was assumed that a service which emphasised responsiveness to locally defined and understood needs would be more effective than one which set national standards and systems for service-provision. This was in part because a locally-responsive service would generate collective commitment among members of families and communities to helping the people in need around them. Also, the model of service was based on local government and local health service provision of service as collectively provided public services.

The symbolic event which commenced the community phase was the implementation of the Seebohm Report (1968) in the Local *Authority Social Services Act, 1970*. This merged the local authority children's departments with welfare and mental health departments, and elements of the then existing local authority health departments, including home help and occupational therapy services. Morever, the service was organised from area offices which served geographical communities, with more concern for local interests. Community work was to be developed to promote public involvement in developing and participating in services within their locality. At the same time, community work was to enhance public involvement in planning decisions, and as part of the attempt to respond to intense problems of deprivation in the inner cities, through the community development projects. Within the social services, the tide of community work receded: most departments did not continue with it.

And yet subsequently it is within the social services that the most substantial commitment to 'community' among local services has continued. This has been in two ways. First, the area structure for delivering services has been enhanced in many parts of the country by a commitment to 'community social work'. Groups of social workers and domiciliary staff work together in very small areas, getting to know local people and working with them to resolve local and personal problems using networks of friends, relatives and neighbours. Promoters of these ideas, particularly Hadley (Hadley and Hatch, 1981), see this as a debureaucratisation or decentralisation which serves people better and connects with their ordinary lives.

Secondly, the personal social services have come to be seen as providing care in the community, while the health service has come to be seen as an institutionally-based service. Such a distinction cannot of course be made about every aspect of these services, since social services departments offer many residential care services often involving fairly substantial institutions, whereas the NHS is based on a widespread network of community health nursing and family doctor services.

With the creation of SSDs in local government and the reorganisation of the NHS in the early 1970s, two empires were created, both with an interest in care and treatment, each separately managed, and both with a role to play. Hunter and Wistow (1987) show that the historic pattern of services and expenditure and the implementation of policies varies between England, Wales and Scotland, affected by continuing differences in approach within the Scottish and Welsh Offices and the DoH, even though the latter often takes a policy lead. The two empires were hard to co-ordinate. The perception of their roles followed the line that the social services were seen as the community alternative to the health service. In order to encourage developments there, rather than in the more expensive and institutionalised health service, governments devised a number of schemes to promote transfer of patients and services from the health to the social services sector. Often, this has involved financial transfers (Hunter and Wistow, 1987).

The first major scheme was *joint finance* which provided for sums of money to be transferred from the NHS budget to the local social services budget to finance projects which would reduce the burden on the health service. It was associated with *joint care planning* (DHSS, 1976, 1977) which required a system of co-operation on the planning of such developments to be set up in each area, allied to general NHS planning mechanisms (Wistow, 1982).

In 1983, the care in the community initiative added central funds to joint finance budgets for a series of experimental schemes designed specifically to set up community projects to enable the discharge of patients from long-stay hospitals (DHSS, 1983a, b).

During this period, a number of changes also took place in the provision of residential care. In most parts of the country, residential care is the most expensive part of social service budgets, and as resources for social services became tighter from the mid-1970s onwards, SSDs increasingly began to look at the possibility of developing other services as an alternative.

In the learning disabilities field, ideas of normalisation began to have a considerable impact on ideology and practice. Within this philosophy it was argued that clients should have a 'normal life', in which they should be provided with care that gave them a lifestyle that contained as many socially-valued aspects of living as possible (Towell, 1988; Brown and Smith, 1992). This began to have effects on other fields, so that in 1988, a survey of the evidence submitted to the Wagner Committee on residential care (Sinclair, 1988) showed that these ideas formed the most widely-held treatment philosophy. While influential, normalisation is a controversial approach, and is considered further in Chapter 6.

The first major moves against residential care were in the child care field, where large and more authoritarian institutions (which also had a poor success rate) were closed down, and there was an increasing emphasis on fostering and various kinds of day provision (Cliffe with Berridge 1991). Similar moves were also evident in services for adults. One important project (the Kent Community Care Scheme, discussed in detail in the next chapter) aimed to provide alternative packages of care to prevent entry into residential care by elderly people.

In other fields, local authorities and interested voluntary groups have continued to expand residential provision for mentally ill people and those with learning difficulties mainly because there is an immense shortage of any kind of provision for these groups. In a sense, the demand for provision with this group of people in need reflects a *housing* problem, which was concealed by warehousing mentally ill people in the larger psychiatric hospitals. However, by the 1980s, particularly encouraged by MIND, the National Association for Mental Health (Bayliss, 1987), there has been an increasing interest in providing various forms of sheltered housing rather than residential care. Mainly, this arises from an interpretation of normalisation which denies the value of anything but 'normal' environments, even where a good deal of care is required. There are fears that institutionalising environments might be recreated on a smaller scale in the community.

Financial restraints on local authorities made it increasingly difficult to increase domiciliary provision for elderly people. The number of elderly people in the population has increased, both absolutely and as a proportion of the population, and this has led to the perception within health and social services that services are not growing fast enough to provide for them.

This problem was relieved somewhat in the early 1980s by a series of events (see Land, 1988, for an account of these) which led to a change in the system of social security benefits so that fairly generous allowances became available to people receiving social security to pay the cost of residential care. There was, however, one major condition – such allowances were only available to people in private and voluntary homes, not those in local authority homes. Availability of residential care allowances made it possible for the first time for a large number of people on social security to afford residential care. It also provided financial incentives for the growth of a private sector of residential care, now the largest provider of residential care beds for elderly people.

The rush to reform in the 1980s

All these changes set the stage for the events leading to the community care reforms embodied in the 1990 Act. The process of development can be seen in a series of reports which progressively refined and defined the problem at issue, and came up with solutions. This process is set out in summary form in Table 2.2.

The ball was set rolling by a report of the House of Commons Select Committee on the Social Services (1985) which criticised the failure to make progress on community care because of these uncertainties, conflicts in policy and particularly financial confusions and pressures. It drew attention to accusations that many people were being discharged from mental hospitals without adequate care after they left.

Following this, the Audit Commission, which carries out investigations of the cost-effectiveness with which government performs its duties, mounted a study of community care and published a report (Audit Commission, 1986) which showed the extent of the failure to implement community care policies consistently throughout the country, and in particular drew attention to the *perverse incentives* within the social security system to encourage people to enter residential care at the cost of central government funding, while com-

Table 2.2 *The development of the 1990 community care reforms*

	Community care	Other developments	Residential care
1982		Barclay Report on the roles and task of social workers published	
1985	House of Commons Select Committee Report on Community Care with special reference to the Mentally Handicapped		
1986	Audit Commission Report 'Making a Reality of Community Care' published	Cumberlege Report 'Neighbourhood Nursing – a Focus for Care' published	Wagner Committee (the independent review of residential care) established
	Griffiths Review of community care policy established	Kent Community Care scheme research published by PSSRU	York (SPRU) residential care assessment research commissioned by DHSS
1987			Firth Report published
1988	Griffiths Report 'Community Care: Agenda for Action' published		Wagner Report 'Residential Care – a Positive Choice' published
1989	Community care White Paper 'Caring for People' published		
1990	*National Health Service and Community Care Act, 1990* enacted		
1991	Policy guidance 'Community Care in the Next Decade and Beyond' published by the Department of Health (DoH)		
1992	Guidance on care management published 'Care Management and Assessment' – managers', practitioners' and summary guides		
1993	Implementation of 'care management' in local authorities		

munity care which should often be cheaper was held back by controls on local government funding.

The government, severely embarassed, immediately announced a further study by Sir Roy Griffiths to identify ways of resolving these problems. His was to be a personal report, from a trusted advisor borrowed from the private sector, although there was a small advisory committee of people knowledgeable about the field. Griffiths had previously been responsible for an important report on the management of the health service (DHSS, 1983c), which led to the replacement of consensus management by a multi-disciplinary team in each health district with the general management system in which appointed managers had full executive control of particular services. Although, this previous work was unconnected to community care, it was the beginning of a series of reforms in the health service which created a new environment of health care for the 1990s, and this provides an important organisational context for community care. Hunter (1994) argues that community care is the missing part in the jigsaw of health provision, forcing health authorities to be involved in it. He also identifies the importance of consumer involvement as a restraint on professional control in the health service, and the development of markets as a way of making provision more cost-effective and less variable in quality, as policy aspects of the government's management approach which are shared by health and community care reforms.

While this was going on, the DHSS commissioned the National Institute for Social Work to undertake an independent review of residential care, in response to signs of growing difficulties and low morale in this sector, and because the Barclay Report (1982) on the role and tasks of social workers had not adequately covered this field of work. This group, chaired by Lady Wagner, began work in mid-1986, and quickly arrived at the view that residential care must be seen in the context of the whole field of community provision. When Sir Roy Griffiths's review began, a certain degree of negotiation took place between these overlapping studies.

The next report to come out was from a committee chaired by Mrs Joan Firth (1987). This had been set up during 1986, at the request of the association which represent the local authorities, to explore the problems that were beginning to arise over the financing of residential care. Probably reflecting its heavy local authority representation, the committee recommended that local authorities should have the responsibility for planning community care and residential services in their areas, and should assess need before admission to social services facilities whichever sector they were in.

At the same time, the Cumberlege Report (1986) (chaired by a leading Conservative local politician, demonstrating that the points of view expressed are likely to have a strong influence on government policy) on community nursing proposed a new structure for neighbourhood nursing services which linked various separate provision into a unified 'area office' with links to but separate from general practice. This reflects concerns about the need for an increasing community focus in the health service. Even though these ideas were not implemented, the Report demonstrates how an alternative base to that of the social services for implementing community care policy was, and could be again, easily possible (Payne, 1987).

The next report to emerge, by a short head, was the report of the Wagner Committee on residential care (1988). The main focus of its approach was that people should not be forced to enter residential care in order to receive services which could be delivered in their own homes. So, residential care should always be the best alternative for them – a positive choice over which the consumer of the services should have as much control as possible. The corollary of this principle is that residential care must always be part of a range of alternatives between which there would be free choice. More information would, according to the Committee's recommendations, be made publicly available about the alternatives.

One element of the Committee's approach (influenced by the Kent Community Care Project, see Chapter 3) is the idea of packages of care which would be devised by a 'nominated social worker' who would be specially trained for this task. The inclusion of this major aspect of post-Griffiths community care policy in this Report on residential care practice and policy as a 'social work' innovation illustrates the close relationship developments in social work practice and community care policy.

Shortly after the Wagner Report, the Griffiths Report (1988) was published. This also stressed the use of case management to create packages of care. Greater emphasis on private, voluntary and informal care was proposed. A controversial aspect of the recommendation was the proposal, similar to the Firth and Wagner recommendations, that local authorities should play a major part in planning and organising community care services in their locality. Generally, the government sought to avoid adding to local authority responsibilities – first, because this tended to increase the overall level of public expenditure in ways which are not easy to control and the government had a policy of maintaining a low level of public expenditure; secondly, because local authorities with political control other than by the Conservative Party are often able to implement policies opposed to central government's view; and thirdly, because as a matter of philosophy, the government preferred non-state options for the provision of services. This preference had not yet been evident in the social services sector, but the success of private residential care showed that it was practicable if a suitable means of finance and management could be found.

After this flurry of reports, all went quiet. The future of community care was to be linked to a major reform of the health service which was being planned, and it was said that the government was seeking to avoid giving local authorities the lead role in providing community care services, consistent with its established approach of reducing the political influence and financial costs of local government. Lobbying from local authority interests and private sector residential care went on.

A year later, in 1989, the government published proposals for the reform of the health service (DoH, 1989a) and associated with it proposals for the community care reforms (DoH, 1989b). Its implementation of the Griffiths Report invoked three major developments:

- local authorities as the lead planning body for community care;
- the purchaser–provider split; and
- the introduction of case (soon to be called 'care') management as the organising principle of the service.

The process which this implies is set out in Figure 2.1. The assumption is of a shared planning process leading to a 'Community Care Plan' for the locality. This process is managed by the local authority (usually the social services department), bringing together a network of providers, in private, voluntary or independent sectors, or public services directly or indirectly managed by the local authority. Representatives of service users and their carers should also participate. The local authority, or the planning consortium, 'contracts' with providers to offer services to the system available

Figure 2.1 *Community care relationships*

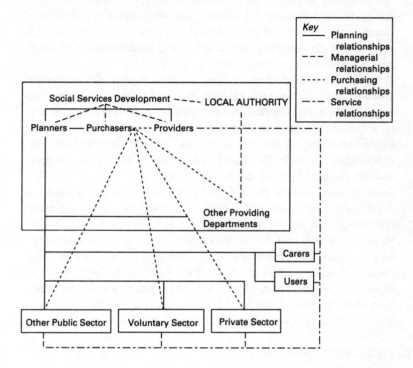

in the area. The local authority (usually), a separate agency or a multi-disciplinary consortium of providers offers a care management service, which 'purchases' a combination of services in each individual case, enabling people in need of services to receive a package of services selected from the range available. Providers within the local authority and other agencies then engage directly with service users and their carers in providing services in accordance with the care plan, monitored by the care manager in the provider part of the social services department.

Although for the future of community care, the primary interest must be in these developments, it is useful to be aware of related changes in the health service, introduced by the same legislation. This is important because, together with the general management reforms of the 1980s, these provide a context within which the health service, one of the partners in community care in any particular area, must operate. Also changes in the health service indicate the direction and import of government thinking in a parallel service, giving us the opportunity to examine the philosophical and political direction of overall policy – although it is important not to impute a co-ordinating intention from coincidental similarities of approach which derive from general philosophical trends.

The basic element of the reforms are the creation of a purchaser–provider split within the health service, as well as in community care. Parts of the health service, previously administered through local health authorities, may become independent 'health care trusts', which then compete on price and quality of service with each other to provide services to the health authorities for their areas, or more widely. Patients are paid for by the health authority, which makes contracts with various trusts for services. If it gets a better offer, it might go to the trust in the next town for, say, geriatrics, while remaining with the trust in this town for paediatrics. Block contracts are established for a certain level of service in each year. This has been further complicated by making arrangements for large groups of general practitioners (family doctors) to become 'fund-holders'. These may also choose and pay for services to which they refer their patients, who may follow a different route from their neighbour who uses the health authority's contracts.

The individual phase

As the *NHS&CCA* passed into law in 1990, the Department of Health (which had been separated from social security in 1989) issued policy guidance (DoH, 1990) on the long-term development of community care services which set the system upon which local authorities worked, and in 1991, the Social Services Inspectorate (SSI) and Scottish Social Work Services Group (SWSG) published detailed guidance on the implementation of care management (SSI/ SWSG, 1991a, b and c). The basic pattern was as proposed in the Griffiths Report, and as set out in Figure 2.1 above; the detail of the guidance is considered below in Chapter 3. I want to consider here the argument that the system which has been set up represents a movement away from commitment to community towards a philosophy of individualisation.

Post-Griffiths community care policy individualises in two ways. First it seeks to divide up a structure of service provision and fragment it, so that each service or location becomes relatively isolated and in some ways in competition with other services. This produces a pattern of services similar to that in the reformed health service, as discussed above. For the government, there is a degree of contradiction, because although the intention of competition is to drive down the cost, and potentially improve the quality, of provision by encouraging the availability of providers who will offer the service more cheaply than the traditional local authority service, it does not wish to increase the cost of the system as a whole by having too much surplus provision, which would arise if many providers were maintained in existence to continue the competitive process. Therefore, it maintains an element of planning in the system, through the local authority-led planning and contracting system.

Under the 'community-collective' assumption, an emphasis is placed on public service collective provision, co-ordinated through major public providers of service in the health and social services authorities. The 'purchaser–provider' split seeks to put local authority providers in much the same position as other contractors, but the extent and importance of their existing provision in most local authority areas usually means that they are dominant providers, especially if voluntary and private providers are not well co-ordinated. Therefore, the government has required a high proportion (85% at the time of writing) of purchased provision to be in the independent sector. Local authorities have in many places dealt with this requirement by establishing major elements of their service as independent, not-for-profit bodies. There are legal restrictions which prevent these bodies from being too closely controlled by councillors or officers from the local authority.

The second form of individualisation is that services in the post-Griffiths world are supposed to be organised around the person who needs them, rather than based on a set range of services – they are 'needs-led' rather than 'service-led'. This means that the needs of the individual become the focus of how services are organised, and makes it more difficult to see services as an overall set of provision. The advantage of this is that service users are not forced into a straitjacket set by the present organisation of services. The disadvantage is that it removes any certainty that services which are available will be taken up, so that managers of services cannot know how many vacancies they will have, and so may not know whether they can finance their service as a whole.

The assumption of competition is that service providers with vacancies will compete on grounds of quality which will attract users (or people such as care managers working on behalf of users) to them. However, providers might prefer or be forced to compete on price, and, as we saw in the last chapter, users and care managers may well have to accept this, if the finance available to users or in the system is insufficient. Also, competition assumes that there is a full range of competing services equally available to each potential user, but this is usually not so. For example, a user might prefer a day centre which is not very good but is close to home to a better one which requires transport.

Community care will, then, consist of a managed market; in many places it will be a highly managed market, because the choice of providers and types of service realistically available to any individual user may well be severely restricted. The management will not all be provided at the planning and contracting level, because the care manager will, at the individual level, probably also be following policies. Such policies might come from their own preferences or from their agency's requirements of or limitations on them.

These opportunities for managing the market in community care are likely to lead to wide variations in how competition works at the local level. There might be a fairly free market in some areas, where there is a political commitment to competition, or there are strong competitive pressures. Such pressures might include a traditional reliance on the voluntary sector for many services, an active and good-quality private sector or a wish to reduce the reliance on public services. In other areas, the possibilities for management of the system and the absence of competitive pressures might ensure the continued dominance of local authority provision, whether directly, or through voluntary or private sector organisations which are heavily influenced by the local authority.

The system in which a social worker or care manager works will have a crucial effect on the reality of alternatives available. The fact that this will be so suggests that workers will need to make judgements about the kind of service that they wish to participate in, and the approach which will be most acceptable to them in their practice. However, the pressures towards individualisation will still be present.

(1) The first of these is the requirement for *assessment* as a funda-

mental basis for providing community care services. This is integral to the DoH guidelines. It means that each service user must have an individual assessment of their needs which must inform him or her of what is provided (hence the term: 'needs-led' services). To some extent, it appears that the user will be able to use the assessment to press the care manager to meet that individualised statement of their needs.

(2) Even where the local authority remains strongly in control, the policy requirement to separate providers from purchasers, and political and financial pressures to privatise local authority services, or use a high proportion of independent providers, must lead to increasing fragmentation of service.

(3) The political imperative to make information about choices available to users and their advisers is likely to increase pressure to deliver the choices which the system increasingly assumes, and which will be welcome to users and their relatives.

(4) There is an underlying value within social work to 'individualise' clients, and where social work has a strong influence on how an agency works, this value base will tend to underline the policy pressures.

(5) Community care assessments are likely to be more comprehensive and flexible than previous assessments for particular services, so they are likely to throw up a more complex pattern of needs to be met. This will tend to work against routine solutions, at least in more complicated cases. At the outset, this has not happened in many places, because of the pressure to assess clients for private sector residential care which was not present before. The opportunity of greater flexibility may be lost if this initial pattern hardens into conventional practice.

The community care services which have emerged from the post-Griffiths reforms of the early 1990s are likely to vary in the extent to which they recognise the competitive individualised ethos which appears to lie behind them: there will be considerable opportunities for local authorities to manage the market. None the less, there are pressures on all sides to maintain the movement towards individualised, needs-led services, so one of the issues which will face workers in the system will be how to enable users of the services to gain benefit from the choices which this might offer them, and to limit the ill-effects of the problems which might arise.

Social work practice, therefore, lies at the centre of the post-Griffiths community care system. The ideas which have led to the reaction against institutional care have been the basis, as we have seen, for the development of 'community'-oriented services throughout the twentieth century. This has led to the growth and development of social work and the social services. The individualising aspect of post-Griffiths policy emphasises how important the personal aspect of care will become. In practice, this will be implemented, or not, at the ground level by successful application of social work skills within each of the three roles identified in Chapter 1: within care management, within community social work/social planning and within therapeutic social work/counselling.

We can also see that this policy brings up to date three historic objectives within community care:

- the discharge of mentally ill people and people with learning disabilities from long-stay hospitals and avoidance of any substantial renewal of the long-stay population of such hospitals;
- the rationalisation of social services, social security and health care systems to avoid the perverse incentives of the 1980s, and to promote a mixed economy of care following the government's management approach; and
- the more diffuse aim of creating a form of care in which people needing long-term care will gain flexibility, independence and support while still living in their own homes surrounded by informal carers from among their relatives and friends.

We shall look again at these historic objectives at the end of Chapter 9, as part of the process of looking forward to the possible achievements and hopes for community care in the 1990s and the early twenty-first century.

Implementing policy objectives through interpersonal work with the most disadvantaged and oppressed has always been the role of social work. The remainder of this book seeks to explore how post-Griffiths community care policy sees social work operating in this context, and the kind of social work practice which might contribute to these objectives.

3

Care Management and Social Work

The practice of care management is central to the implementation of the 1990s community care policy. The purpose of this chapter is to examine the ideas contained in 'care management' to see how these are being implemented in community care practice and to relate care management to social work practice. Two main approaches to care management exist. One is the 'social care entrepreneurship' approach developed from American 'case management' and introduced into the UK primarily through the influence of the Kent Community Care Project. Since this was the model adopted by the DoH in its guidance, it is the primary focus of this chapter. The second is the 'service brokerage' approach, developed from Canadian models, and used in the UK in more multi-disciplinary, user-oriented projects. These focus on getting co-operation between services and encouraging service users to plan and make their own demands. Doria Pilling (1992) has developed a further distinction between service brokerage and multi-disciplinary care management; this latter form focuses on organising a multi-disciplinary team, particularly using a 'keyworker'. This is introduced in the latter part of this chapter to offer comparisons with the model adopted by the DoH, and features of care management relevant to both models are explored.

The latter part of this chapter also explores how the American case management model has been transmuted into the official care management model promoted by the DoH. Early experiments in implementation identify some of the difficulties and possibilities for social work practice in care management.

The aim of the first part of this chapter is to show how the American context for the formation of 'case management' produced a set of ideas that was implemented in the UK for different purposes. When these ideas were implemented within community care policy, they were expanded and formalised into a concept of 'care management', and attempts were made to distinguish this concept from previously existing social work practice. I argue that, even though there are new aspects of care management, the idea still contains and requires the use of important social work skills which are the focus of this book. In the USA, some writers regard it as a form or implementation of social work, rather than as something separate. We should distinguish care management from social work, therefore, but we should also see the links.

Figure 3.1 provides an overview of the main influences on the concept of care management as it is being implemented in community care policy. The central influence of the PSSRU (the Personal Social Services Research Unit of the University of Kent) is because of its implementation of the American concept of case management initially in the Kent Community Care Scheme. PSSRU also had the research contract for evaluating the government's early 1980 experiments in de-institutionalisation within the 'Care in the Community' Programme. Whereas this was at first a separate programme, the ideas being developed in PSSRU began to influence the outcomes of this work too, and further experiments developed, testing and expanding these concepts elsewhere. This experience then became an important influence on the DoH guidance to practitioners and managers on the implementation of the 1990 Act.

The development and more detailed analysis of these ideas is the main focus of this chapter.

American 'case management'

American 'case management' developed in the context of American social services where hospitals, community facilities and social work agencies are typically relatively unco-ordinated, independent institutions, often in what in the UK would be the voluntary or private sectors. When, as with everywhere else in the world, the professional and political moves to shift care from institutions to community provision became significant in the 1970s and 1980s,

Figure 3.1 *Development of care management concepts*

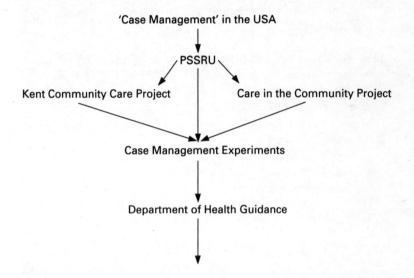

'Case Management' in the USA

PSSRU

Kent Community Care Project   Care in the Community Project

Case Management Experiments

Department of Health Guidance

processes were required for co-ordinating this provision. Generally, public welfare services are less predominant in their locality than in the UK, so it was not assumed that these would come from statutory services, and the method of case management became the crucial concept, rather than any widespread acceptance of an organisational structure.

Much of the early work emphasised the removal of mentally ill people from hospitals to the community and was '. . . viewed as a means of overcoming the complexity and fragmentation of our service system and of reaching the inadequately served chronically and severely disabled population' (Miller, 1983). In Miller's comment, here, we see another important aspect of case management: it is concerned to seek out people who are hard to find in the population.

The techniques spread to other related services, and an extensive survey by Weil *et al.* (1985) describes them in use among children, elderly people and their families, and people with learning difficulties and physical disabilities as well as mentally ill people. These authors define case management as a set of logical steps and a process of interaction within a service network which assure that a client receives needed services in a supportive, effective, efficient and cost-effective manner. (Weil and Karls, 1985, p. 2)

They emphasise accountability within a complex set of services in their use of words such as 'assure' 'effective' and 'efficient', but also focus on personal relationship in case management with phrases such as 'process of interaction' and 'supportive . . . manner'.

Moxley (1989) in a recent account of American case management practice defines it as:

a client-level strategy for promoting the coordination of human services, opportunities, or benefits. The major outcomes . . . are: (1) the integration of services across a cluster of organisations . . .; and (2) achieving continuity of care. (Moxley, 1989, p. 11)

The importance given here to 'client-level' emphasises that even work between organisations and services concerns the client's personal needs, and should be worked on at that level, not as a managerial or bureaucratic task.

American case management may be undertaken from a variety of organisational bases and by people occupying a number of different roles. Weil (1985) analyses a variety of roles within which it is possible to undertake case management:

- generalist service-broker (for example, social services area team intake worker)
- primary therapist (for example, social services long-term or hospital social worker; family therapist)
- interdisciplinary team (for example, community mental handicap or health team)
- comprehensive service centre (for example, health centre with attached social workers)
- family (for example, family members of the person needing care)
- supportive care manager (for example, home care organiser)
- volunteer (for example, neighbour, volunteer from local care service).

The 'logical steps' (as Weil and Karls, 1985, put it) of case management are variously defined, and Table 3.1 sets out three differ-

Table 3.1 *Formulations of the components of American case management and British care management*

Steinberg and Carter (1983)	Weil (1985)	Moxley (1989)	DoH (1991)
case finding (that is, identifying all potential clients with a set of criteria)	client identification and outreach		publishing determining level of assessment (screening)
assessment	individual assessment and diagnosis	assessment	needs assessment
goal setting and services planning	service planning and resource identification	planning	care planning
care plan implementation	linking clients to needed services service implementation and co-ordination	intervention	implementing care plan
monitoring	monitoring service delivery advocacy evaluation	monitoring evaluation	monitoring reviewing

ent formulations, comparing them with the eventual official British formulation.

The two slightly earlier accounts stress the importance of searching out possible clients who are not identified. The more pragmatic Moxley moves straight on to assessment; Renshaw (1988) suggests that referral and case-finding tend to be less important where the service is concerned with an already identified group of service users, such as people being discharged from long-stay hospital. Otherwise, these analyses of the components of case management are similar. Weil is alone in including advocacy on behalf of service users within the care system after carrying out initial monitoring, although in alternative conceptualisations of case management and in the definition of social work, this is an important function. Also important is the distinction drawn by Weil and by Moxley between monitoring (periodically checking that the planned services are co-ordinating well) and evaluation (a more considered review of the success of the outcomes after the process has been carried out).

Steinberg and Carter (1983) identify what they consider to be the crucial features of a case management system (as opposed to the definition and practice of case management which we have been discussing so far). In their view, the service delivery system has to offer:

- *comprehensiveness* – there has to be a sufficiently diverse range of services to provide a wide range of options for service users
- *continuity* – so that users' movements through the system are co-ordinated;
- *adequacy* – there has to be a big enough supply of each option to enable it to be provided when required (so there will be some redundancy and a level of vacancies in the system);
- *quality* – the service has to meet performance standards, and the standards should be acceptable to the users and (often) their relatives and carers.

This brief account indicates some of the important features of case management as it had grown up in the USA by the late 1980s. Throughout, we can see the importance given to personal relationships and direct work with the client; as originally conceived, then, this activity is very much like an implementation of social work. Huxley (1991) evaluated 14 research studies of its effectiveness, carried out between 1985 and 1990, and identifies three characteristics of effective services for mentally ill people: they are specific about

- objectives
- the case management model used
- the target group of service users.

He proposes, based on unpublished research in services in Salford and Derby in the UK, that attempts to adapt existing services to case management or to add elements of case management to existing services have not proved effective, and that specifically designed and targeted services are likely to be more successful. Schorr (1992, p. 38), an American reviewing British developments in the personal social services, comments that his impression is that 'in the United States, at any rate,... failure of care management is epidemic in Departments of Human Services – for lack of adequate funding, to begin with, so that one never gets to the question of whether the concept is sound'.

Importing case management

The American concept of case management was imported into the UK through the crucial agency of the PSSRU in its work first on the Kent Community Care scheme and then later. To see how it has been adapted through that process it is necessary to review in some detail that major project and some of the PSSRU's other work.

The 'production of welfare approach'

The PSSRU has a fundamental theoretical approach, called 'the production of welfare' approach, which imports into social policy thinking some of the ideas of micro-economics. In summary, the idea is that the welfare of individuals is 'produced' through the interaction of a variety of 'inputs' such as the efforts of individuals with social and personal needs, their personalities and attitudes, the work of service providers, money and facilities provided by specialist welfare services, and so on. These inputs interact with each other in a social environment which affects how the interaction takes place, and this produces a welfare 'outcome', which can be evaluated according to the extent to which it meets the needs of the person whose welfare we are concerned with. The production of welfare approach studies inputs and how they interact, and evaluates the welfare outcomes: both intermediate outcomes (such as the kinds of services provided) and the final outcomes (such as costs, and the effects on both the community and the client group for whom services were provided).

The approach proposes that by understanding human (and other) aspects of the interaction, you can begin to understand what factors will lead inputs to produce valued outcomes, and what factors lead to unsatisfactory outcomes. Case (care) management is an example of looking at the process of what goes on in the interaction

of inputs and identifying a model of that process – case (care) management – which seems to be particularly effective. While PSSRU
writers claim the importance of these factors (see for example, Davies
and Knapp, 1988, pp. 2–3), much of their work (and this is increasingly so in their work on the implementation of the community
care reforms) concentrates on costing and rather underrates other
aspects.

This approach appears powerful for the analysis of community
care. It gives a central role to costs, and we saw in Chapters 1 and
2 how important cost containment is in the history and policy debate about community care. Also, it focuses on understanding and
analysing how services might substitute for one another, and provides a model for assessing the cost and outcome consequences of
substituting one service for another. This, then, was the approach
which the PSSRU had when it came to experiment in the late 1970s
with a community care service in Kent.

The Kent Community Care Project

The main account of this project is contained in Davies and Challis
(1986); page references given below are to that book, unless otherwise stated.

The project (pp. 227–37) involved a specialist team of workers
in a typical generic area team, which moved later to a short-stay
home for elderly people. Its job was to provide additional or alternative care for elderly people who would otherwise be very likely to
go into residential care. This was a clear and limited focus for its
work, which Huxley's (1991) comments, discussed above, suggest
would provide the best basis for effective case management. The
team had authority to plan *and implement* innovative arrangements
over most of the system of care. Early on they spent time building
links with local services and the area team, both as part of a process of 'case-finding and screening' and to link with services that
they might call on. When they started, they were typical of the
less-qualified but experienced people often found in adult teams at
the time. Clients were found from the caseload of the area team,
the existing waiting list for residential care and the home help
caseload. This was a very low proportion of the cases where work
was being done by the department; for example, very few home
help cases who were not already on the residential care waiting list

were considered sufficiently needy. It was found that a more personal referral system by discussion (rather than form-based) produces more and more suitable referrals. The workers had small caseloads, relative to other workers in the team.

Some features of the team's work sought to strengthen case management and to develop an innovative approach to community care (pp. 8–13). First, control of a budget was delegated, and everything actually or notionally charged against it, so that workers could be aware of the relative costs of decisions they were making. The initial budget for each client was two-thirds of the cost of a residential care home place (although more could be sought with management approval), so that expenditure was not concentrated on a few cases. Since the screening criteria and objectives of the project concerned people at serious risk of admission to residential care, this provision also reduced potential costs to the department, since if the community care scheme worked the number of people needing residential care would be reduced.

Secondly, new procedures were to be introduced, and from this new, more creative and flexible conventions in providing community care services would be developed, which would not be limited by regulations and procedures, Flexibility and resourcefulness would be enhanced by teamwork and debate within and between teams.

Thirdly, there would be a team of experienced workers, whose skills would command confidence from local services, and who would have a manageable caseload to enable them to do thoroughly all the necessary work in each case. Thus, each worker would be clearly responsible for everything that happened with a particular case, and their success in creating and managing a network of care for their client would be transparent to client, carers and community. Accountability was enhanced by recording and case review systems which provided clear statements of clients' problems and needs and ensured that flexible budgets were used properly.

After setting up and the case finding, referral and screening phase, the project used the following stages of case management: assessment, care planning, service arrangement and monitoring (pp. 235–64). These stages are very similar to the various American formulations in Table 3.1, demonstrating how the American model has been imported.

In the *assessment* phase, several visits were required for a detailed initial assessment, and the extent of the assessment and the low caseloads permitted strong influence on the assessment by carers and clients themselves and by other workers and helpers. Controlling the budget gave case managers an incentive to carry out the assessment more carefully, because they had the capacity to respond to the variations in clients' needs that they could identify.

In the *service arrangement* phase, workers spent most of their time on continuing contacts with their clients, after care packages had been arranged. Among their important activities were: making help that clients needed acceptable to them, helping clients cope with loss of a close carer or spouse, meeting the personal and information needs of informal carers and mobilising and co-ordinating services to the client from different services. The study compared the seven services most frequently received by clients before and after joining the project. The importance of reliance on the home help service and aids for helping with disability was reduced (but still important) whereas the provision of social work help increased in importance and help from informal carers appeared from nowhere. Though informal care was the major new development, the project, as with American case management, emphasised the value of social work within case management.

One of the most important aspects of service introduced by the project to the area was the recruitment of neighbours, relatives and other informal carers, paid small allowances or expenses to take up an important role in providing services. A pool of helpers was recruited in advance, and was added to in particular cases; helpers were then matched to people needing help and supported in providing it. An important task was to avoid exploitation of carers, often by themselves in their commitment to help. Qureshi *et al.* (1989) undertook a study of the role of and effects on the helpers in the project. Most helpers were middle-aged women; some unemployed or disabled men were recruited. Half of the helpers were working class, with a record of work in service and clerical jobs; unusually for such projects younger women with children were recruited. This may be a result of the payment made. The early motivations of helpers were:

- having time to spare, needing stimulation, getting away from family problems and needing social contacts
- wish for material gain, particularly where they needed flexible working arrangements

- need for being useful, for more independence, to make a contribution to society
- a desire to help others.

Most helpers had their wishes met, but the relationships with individual clients became more important as they gained experience. Most of those who left the project did so for personal reasons, particularly that helping was not for them. Those who stayed acquired a personal commitment to their clients, but payment was important where the client or the work was difficult. Qureshi *et al.* (1989) developed a theory that helping was characterised by social, economic and altruistic *exchanges* between helpers, clients and the project. The practice implication of this is that workers need to ensure that the social benefits, pay and personal satisfaction gained by helpers matches the extent and difficulty of their input to caring. Also, the element of 'exchange' suggests the importance of respecting and listening to helper and informal carers.

Monitoring was carried out by the workers continuously, as they maintained their regular contact with service-providers, clients, carers and helpers providing the packages of care.

In evaluating the *outcomes* of the project, the researchers looked at the welfare of clients and carers (pp. 369–94) and cost comparisons (pp. 401–507). They matched similar pairs of clients; one of each pair received the project service, the other did not. In summary, significantly fewer elderly people in the project went into residential care; significantly fewer died; their physical abilities declined less. It may have been that the service delayed rather than prevented such progression to more intensive services. They also used other institutional facilities (for example, geriatric day hospital) less. They felt happier and thought that they had an improved quality of care. Informal carers experienced significantly less mental stress, and were not demotivated by the extra support given; they did not reduce their caring activities. This finding is important because of the suggestion from right-wing thinkers that the more official service is provided, the less informal care will be offered; in the case of this project, this appears not to be so. Close, confiding relationships developed between elderly people, carers and workers on the project and this meant that significantly more than the matched group had someone in whom they could confide. In this sense, their personal relationships improved.

In assessing costs, the researchers compared the costs of the community care service against the standard provision in social services departments (pp. 472–3). Broadly, they showed that the community care service tended to allocate resources rationally according to the level of dependency, unaffected by how demanding carers or clients were, whereas standard provision often perversely allocates more resources to those with less strong needs, because of demands made by carers or clients. In general, costs are lower for community care, and there was no break-even point where community care became more expensive. Community care was particularly cost-effective where it allowed extensive support to be given at an early stage to elderly people with considerable physical or mental infirmity; it avoided very expensive services at a crisis level later on.

Community care saved most money for the health service from services for very frail client groups. However, it was cost-effective for virtually all client groups with lower levels of dependency, since if they received inappropriate residential care, there was a considerable gap between the cost of this and the fairly insignificant costs of the level of community care they needed. Conversely, we need to be cautious in saying that more co-ordinated delivery of home services will meet the needs of very dependent groups. Askham and Thompson (1990) studied a similar scheme for dementia sufferers, who survived longer when in care rather than in the community. Doria Pilling (1992) surmises, in comparing this project with the Kent project, that the level of home care for very demented elderly people makes no difference to whether they can stay at home.

These findings suggest that community care needs to concentrate on identifying those with lower levels of need who would otherwise end up in residential care, since this would lead to improvements in their quality and length of life, make the greatest cost savings and make available more residential care places for those with greater disabilities. Moreover, the community care project workers showed that they could actually differentiate between levels of dependency and respond with appropriate services, without putting expensive services where they were not needed.

Care in the Community and other PSSRU projects

The Kent project was undertaken in a suburban retirement area, and the PSSRU applied similar techniques with largely similar results to urban areas, in Gateshead (Challis *et al.*, 1988; Challis *et al.*, 1990) and Darlington (Challis *et al.*, 1989). However, the Care in the Community demonstration programme, which included the Darlington project, also contributed through PSSRU to developing case management concepts in the UK.

'Care in the Community' was launched in 1983, by the government, to fund a number of pilot projects to help long-stay patients leave hospital with the aim of demonstrating and encouraging the deinstitutionalisation of long-term hospital care (Renshaw *et al.*, 1989). It is an interesting comment on the government's priorities that the subtitle of an early document (DHSS, 1981) referred to 'moving resources' rather than referring to care arrangements. Authorities were encouraged to continue experimentation. This possibility was enhanced by the circular establishing the pilot projects (DHSS, 1983b). Guidance was issued at the same time (DHSS, 1983a), encouraging the participation of voluntary organisations, and acceptance of projects encouraged such participation – an early sign of the government's interest in promoting a wider range of care providers.

Most projects eventually approved were for mentally ill people or people with learning difficulties, but there were also projects for young people with multiple difficulties, for people with physical disabilities, for elderly, physically frail people and elderly people with mental health problems (Knapp *et al.*, 1990, 1992, p. 10).

These projects, therefore, were concerned with community care for people leaving an institution, rather than the preventive approach of the Kent project: they approached community care from the opposite end of the spectrum, and so they provide a useful comparison with the Kent project. They were also much more strongly concerned with the creation of new facilities for the patients, and in particular with their housing. This was not so much of an issue with the Kent project; consequently, the material on case management (the focus of this chapter) was more limited. It was not, for example, strongly in evidence in an early set of papers from participants in the project (Cambridge and Knapp, 1988). To some extent, the importance given to this technique in the final reports probably reflects the PSSRU's increasing influence in formulating ideas of case management during the period that the projects were working. It may also reflect a conceptualisation of a variety of different developments in the original projects into a more flexible, looser account of case management, expanding on the ideas derived from the Kent scheme.

These projects provided an opportunity to evaluate the use of case management techniques with a range of different client groups, and particularly with mentally ill people, who are at the centre of debate about deinstitutionalisation policies. The project found (Challis *et al.*, 1990, pp. 17–20; Knapp *et al.*, 1992, pp. 206–34) that a variety of case management models was used within what had become the standard PSSRU statement of the core tasks of case management:

● case finding and referral
● assessment and selection
● care planning and service packaging
● monitoring and assessment, and
● case closure.

With these client groups, the problems at *referral and selection* stage were often of defining selection criteria to identify suitable clients from a larger number of potential service users. Systems differed, but the process usually included gathering information from surveys of patients and referrals from community or hospital staff leading to a mechanism for an initial decision about potential suitability for continued stay in hospital or for resettlement. Then, there was a multi-disciplinary *assessment*, and the patient was referred to the project, which collected more detailed information about the patient relevant to the project's work, consulted with the client and others involved and developed a programme plan for resettlement.

At the *care planning* stage, each project had a system for creating an individual plan, often called an 'individual programme plan'. These led to regular reviews and reassessments throughout the time that rehabilitation work was going on.

Delivering services was usually conceived as a team activity, because it encouraged multi-disciplinary work (although this was sometimes not very effectively carried out), developed a democratic management style, encouraged peer support and helped in identifying basic objectives for the project. Relationships with existing community mental handicap and mental health teams were harder to progress. Most schemes had a system of providing a keyworker for each client, similar to the case manager in the Kent project, who maintained personal responsibility for that client's needs and development. There were devolved budgets in only two projects, but most were fairly small projects with a specific budget supplied by the grant, separately from ordinary funding. An emphasis was placed on user involvement in many projects, going beyond keeping them informed and consultation to genuine two-way relationships between clients and case managers. Relatives were also involved in various, usually rather more limited, ways (more limited perhaps, because most were not actively caring for the client, who had usually been in hospital for some time).

The researchers devised a typology of case management arrangements:

- residential social work, where the keyworker was based in a residential or housing setting
- sub-area social services, where a case manager was based in a more generic team
- peripatetic social services, using senior social work staff, some from the area team and some from health service backgrounds
- multi-disciplinary, with a joint health and social services team
- multi-disciplinary teams, solely within the health authority
- quasi-brokerage, using mechanisms such as individualised funding agreements
- semi-independent, where the case manager was a worker with clients outside the statutory sector, although usually with some health and social services involvement through providing funding for individual clients.

To develop case management in these kinds of projects, the researchers proposed that:

- assessment and monitoring procedures needed to be multi-disciplinary and comprehensive in character, offering opportunities for user involvement and representation;
- better accountability and cost consciousness would have been achieved by devolved budgeting;
- peripatetic, multi-disciplinary teams bridged professional and agency divides better than single-agency or residential-based case managers;
- more objective decision-making comes from separating case management from keyworking and service provision, and enables

case managers to advocate more appropriately for their clients, since they are independent of providing the service;
● accountability to both employer and service user was a problem for public sector case managers; independent or semi-independent arrangements were more successful in dealing with this part of the case management role.

Other related concepts and projects

The PSSRU approach to case management was not the only one. Beardshaw and Towell (1990, p. 18) describe it as a form of *'social care entrepreneurship'* in which formal and informal care are interwoven according to individual need by a worker who takes on the role of entrepreneur in getting the system running for the benefit of the client. They contrast this with a *'service brokerage'* approach adopted from Canadian models, where the emphasis is on working with a service user as an advocate to fill gaps in the services identified by the client. Brandon (1989) describes the Community Living Society of Vancouver, one of the originators of this approach. Brokers act as 'travel agents' working with users to identify and share information with users and their families, and help them implement their own vision of a good service for themselves. This clearly places less emphasis on the co-ordination of services and more on the client's own action as part of the process of gaining services. A third model, building on this distinction, is identified by Doria Pilling (1992) who discusses programmes in which a *multi-disciplinary team* is responsible for assessment and developing a care plan for an individual. Often this is delegated to particular members of the team, acting on the team's behalf, although the responsibility is clearly that of the team. This model sometimes explicitly uses a *'keyworker'*.

The term 'keyworker' presents a number of problems. In the *social services*, it tends to refer to co-ordinating relationships between workers involved with clients who are in residential care. The keyworker is a residential worker with particular responsibility for being aware of the needs of a resident. This is necessary because in group care settings individual needs were sometimes lost sight of, and it was easier for the client's fieldworker to have one person to contact within a residential care staff group. The term has sometimes been extended to refer to the person with responsibility for a client at risk (such as a child on the 'at risk' register) so that one identified person is responsible for acting and receiving information.

In the *health care field*, the term 'keyworker' has more often been used for the designated member of a multi-disciplinary team responsible for progress-chasing action required for a patient. Hunter (1988) describes projects of this kind for disability and head injuries teams. Beardshaw and Towell (1990, p. 22) summarise research findings about the difficulties of such schemes. Interprofessional rivalry sometimes inhibits action and gaining resources from different agencies may depend on service managers from outside the team and their own assessment of the case. Different professionals operate in different ways, and the team often defines the task very widely, so that keyworkers have to limit the role in their own way. Both these problems lead to inconsistency in how service is provided. There is also evidence that monitoring long-term clients is difficult if keyworkers also have to work short-term with other clients.

Doria Pilling (1992) provides well-researched accounts of two teams operating brokerage and multi-disciplinary teamwork models. In the following accounts, page numbers refer to her book, unless otherwise stated.

The Camden and Islington project for people with physical disabilities (pp. 81–129) worked from the premise that the user's needs and wishes were the most important basis for deciding on services, and should be separated from service-allocation decisions. The project was widely advertised and sought referrals from potential clients directly. Anyone with a physical disability was accepted. There was an extensive assessment, followed by an agreement with the user, who would then be given information about services that they could approach themselves, or that the worker would negotiate on their behalf. Personal help and counselling was excluded from the case manager's role. A user group formed, and there was advocacy for better services and involvement in decision-making. Eventually, a voluntary organisation with a service development role grew up.

The evaluation showed that about 150 clients were helped, and in spite of its advocacy role (which could have been seen as hostile), was accepted by local services, except for occupational therapists who thought that it helped some clients 'jump the queue' for services. Clients were satisfied with the service and it did seem to improve the range of service offered. Advocacy and co-ordination seemed to support each other: the worker needed well-worked out plans and full information in order to take an advocacy role. The main reason that tasks could not be completed was lack of resources in the services. The fact that the organisation was independent of mainstream services but not seen as in opposition to them, but rather as a resource, seemed to be an effective form of management.

The other disability project researched by Pilling (pp. 133–78) was a multi-disciplinary team based in the health service in two London boroughs, Kensington and Chelsea, and Westminster. Occupational, speech and physio-therapists, together with an administrator and part-time psychologist, were managed by a nurse. Disabled people referred mainly by statutory services had a 'keyworker' appointed, who investigated the history of their involvement with other agencies and then carried out a joint assessment with another member of the team.

The aim was to improve the quality of disabled people's lives by providing information and advice, an assessment and continuing support. However, the team took time to develop its work because its methods were not clearly defined, and this meant that other agencies were unclear about its role. It built up a great deal of knowledge of local resources, and clients valued its expertise and support highly. Service providers in the area were confused, however, about whether its purpose was gathering information about the needs of clients for the benefit of planning, or providing a service to clients. The team saw these roles as integrated, but this was not always evident to outsiders.

Physiotherapists who tended to refer patients but not work jointly with the team were more uncertain about its role than social workers and other local authority staff who worked jointly with it. Many people involved felt that strong leadership and management support was essential to the team developing its role effectively. The fact that the project was placed wholly in the health service was also widely felt to be a disadvantage: a joint project would have worked better.

These projects have a different emphasis within case management from the Kent project. They, and the 'care in the community' projects, offer ways of integrating multi-disciplinary work and of bringing advocacy into practice within community care. Such an emphasis seems to come from the organisational base from which these projects arose and from the fact that they worked with disabled people in the prime of life who sought and demanded greater independence by receiving a wide variety of services, rather than dependent elderly people applying for supportive services from a social services department, or dependent mentally ill people being discharged from long-stay hospitals.

Similar experience grew out of extensive work on multi-disciplinary teamwork in the learning difficulties and mental health field. Projects which have been extensively researched are the community mental handicap teams established widely as a way of co-ordinating health and social services activities, particularly in discharging people with learning difficulties from hospital (see Chapter 6). The All Wales Strategy for people with learning difficulties was an important forerunner in developing these ideas of needs-led multi-disciplinary services (McGrath and Grant, 1992).

Another related concept, *care programming*, has developed within services for mentally abnormal offenders and other mentally ill people who need fairly extensive treatment in hospital. The aims (DoH, 1992a) are similar to those of case management, requiring a full assessment of needs, the appointment of a keyworker who coordinates provision of services and regular review and monitoring of services. Research by Schneider (1993) suggests that most of this work was carried out from a health service base by community psychiatric nurses, and did not involve extensive multi-disciplinary work and meetings. This system was not well integrated into the community care plans of many local authorities. A DoH study (1993e) suggests that developing ideas of care management in SSDs made it difficult to integrate the two systems fully, and that health authorities were having difficulties in the early stages in implementing care programming. Onyett and Davenport (1993) report an experiment in Kent which tried to merge the two approaches. The development of regular clinical review meetings involving community and hospital staff, an integrated computer record system encouraging co-operation and a co-ordinator to develop shared work were the main methods used to overcome difficulties experienced elsewhere.

Formalising care management

Initial application of case management to community care

As a result of the work of the PSSRU in the Kent project, the 'social care entrepreneurship' concept of case management was well-established as an important innovation by the time Griffiths produced his report (1988). He recommended (para 6.6) that

> In cases where a significant level of resources are involved a 'care manager' should be nominated from within the social service authority's staff to oversee the assessment and reassessment function and manage the resulting action.

The virtually simultaneous Wagner Committee Report on residential care recommended:

> Individuals and their families should have available to them the skills of a nominated social worker ... whose primary responsibility is to act as their agent, and who should be trained in the individual assessment of needs and in the imaginative creation of a package of services designed to meet them. (Wagner, 1988, p. 28)

Both of these proposals draw directly on the PSSRU importation of American case management ideas, but they are different in focus. Griffiths is more concerned with case management as a process for managing resources and arranging services effectively. Wagner approaches case management as a means of user involvement in and control of decision-making, and we have seen above how the PSSRU approach to case management also included this approach more strongly as it became more involved in the mental health and learning difficulties services, where advocacy and user involvement has a stronger history. The tension between facilitating resource management and user participation continues to lie within the case management role, in the same way that, as we have seen in Chapters 1 and 2, cost containment and welfare enhancement lie at the heart of the tensions in community care policy and history.

Care Management in the 'Policy Guidance'

The subsequent Policy Guidance (DoH, 1990) finally formalised *care* management as a major part of its requirements of local authorities in implementing the *NHS&CCA, 1990*. Its role would be to

● ensure that available resources would be used effectively

- restore and maintain independence by enabling people to live in the community
- minimise the effects of disability and illness
- treat service users respectfully and provide equal opportunities
- promote individual choice and self-determination, and build on existing strengths and care resources
- promote partnership between users, carers and service providers and organisations representing them.

This reflects the interpersonal focus of American case management, the emphasis on resources developed from the American need for co-ordination, the government's policy objectives and the production of welfare approach of PSSRU, and also the advocacy and user participation perspectives derived from the care in the community project and imported into the social work world from user participation work, particularly in the mental health and learning disabilities fields. At one point (para. 3.17), the Guidance suggests that some users should play a part in their own care management.

However, it also contains certain service objectives and values, such as minimising disability and illness and promoting equal opportunities, which are consistent with case management ideas but seek to use care management to develop wider objectives. This might be a sign of official expectations that care management will be the vehicle for achieving everything, instead of recognising its limited role and acknowledging that promoting policy objectives such as equal opportunities, or more ambitiously, anti-discriminatory work, will require more comprehensive action. The absence of anti-discriminatory perspectives from the PSSRU and other work is partly a consequence of the time and place it was done and partly a result of the focus of the research on costs and management, rather than the individual needs of clients. No doubt the emphasis on self-determination and independence reflects the government's political anxiety about social services making people dependent on the welfare state.

Huxley (1993) attempts to distinguish 'care' from 'case' management, claiming that internationally case management has a long history of use and evaluative research, whereas 'care' management has a less clear provenance, and is more concerned with management tasks in care settings. However, it seems clear that what the DoH is proposing is 'case' management in the conventional sense, and the term 'care' management is being used as a euphemism to avoid treating people as 'cases'.

SSDs are expected by the Policy Guidance to establish care management arrangements and supporting budgetary arrangements (para. 3.57). The Guidance says:

> Care managers should be able to assume some or all of the responsibility for purchasing the services necessary to implement a care plan. Such a devolution of responsibility brings decision-making closer to service users and thus makes it more responsive to their needs . . . It will have its greatest impact where most of the processes involved are carried out by a single care manager who has some measure of responsibility for a devolved budget. (DoH, 1990, pp. 24–5)

The care management systems should be flexible in responding to users' and carers' needs, making a range of options available, intervening only to foster independence or to prevent deterioration, and concentrating on clients with the greatest needs. They will need to work in the context of priority decisions made by the authority's community care plans, but should feed back into those plans the findings from assessments and experience of implementing the care plans. The needs-led approach to case management is seen in the Guidance as having two key aspects: in separating assessment from service provision by focusing on the client's needs and in shifting influence on assessment from providers to purchasers (DoH, 1990, pp. 23–4).

This part of the Guidance contains the first attempts to integrate the idea of care management into the area-wide system of management and planning for community care. Devolved budgets are maintained, which was such an important part of the Kent scheme, and which might well have been lost in the application of a small experimental project to a nation-wide development within bureaucratic local government systems. One reason for its continued life might be the importance within the government's management approach (discussed in Chapter 1) of marketisation, devolution and clarification of responsibility of individual workers.

The process of care management is given as three distinct processes, emphasising user and carer participation:

- assessment (which is given the emphasis of a separate section of the Guidance)
- design of a 'care package'
- implementation and monitoring.

One consequence of this foreshortening of the American and PSSRU models of case management is the increasing emphasis given to assessment and design of the care package, perhaps leading to an assumption that implementation is a fairly routine consequence of the design process. This might have been brought about by the intended split between providing and purchasing service. Since the care manager is seen as part of the purchasing machinery and will have no responsibility for provision, the sophisticated involvement in interpersonal work with clients found in the Kent project and which derives from the centrality of social work to the American and Kent models might well get lost. One of the aims of this book is to mitigate that tendency.

Care plans (creating the package of care), according to the Guidance (p. 27), will include the services to be provided or arranged and the objectives of interventions. A clear set of priorities is defined, moving from the most desirable to the least – for example: support in the service user's own home, moving to more suitable accommodation, moving to another private household, residential, nursing home and long-stay hospital care. This is reflected in the 'community care tariff' assumed in most post-Griffiths policy (see Chapter 5). The possibility of conflicts between the need for cost-effectiveness, users' and carers' preferences and quality of care are noted, and points of disagreement should be recorded.

As well as DoH work, various other local and national experiments and developmental work was undertaken. For example, the Association of Directors of Social Services (ADSS) undertook both conceptual and technical work to develop a more agreed approach to community care. A feature of their document (ADSS/SSI, 1991) is an attempt to create a set of priorities, which indicates managerial thinking about the role of care management, and reflects the acceptance of the 'community care tariff'. Social services resources would be 'targeted' at those in the first three priority groups. Clients who ask or are referred for services are 'screened'. Those who are seen as 'coping' are redirected to other services. Those who are beginning to display problems are given a nominated worker (with a lower level of skill and no control over resources) to prevent deterioration. Care management only comes into play where rehabilitation from care or significant degrees of help are required, or where there is a 'significant risk to life or major injury' (ADSS/SSI, 1991, p. 13). It appears that this involves the worker in more activity, but developing a package of services through a 'care plan' is reserved for a situation in which there is a crisis or serious difficulties involving a 'substantial' risk to life.

This approach is consistent with the case management concept as we have seen it develop in its attempt to reserve care management to a fairly severe situation requiring co-ordination of resources; the stated aim is 'to ensure only those individuals who need specialised help are assessed for services' (ADSS/SSI, 1991, p. 11). It tries to incorporate a view of care management which recognises the resource constraints likely to be felt by social service agencies. It seems, however, to regard 'care management' as mainly a form of social work intervention designed to prevent the need to go forward to develop a full care plan, and keep services 'down the tariff'. Such an approach seems to aim, in traditional local authority fashion, to delay implementing care management in the full sense to as late a stage as possible, probably in order to avoid committing resources. As we have seen, one of the important aspects of care management in the Kent project and others was the capacity to distinguish situations where deterioration was likely and react strongly enough to prevent it. The view of care management as a form of service broking may be included in work at the second and third priority levels; advocacy does not receive a mention.

The 'Care Management and Assessment' guides

The final state of formalisation of care management as part of post-Griffiths community care provision came about with the publication of two guides (and a summary – SSI/SWSG, 1991c) for practitioners (SSI/SWSG, 1991a) and managers (SSI/SWSG, 1991b) in establishing care management and assessment services under the *NHS&CCA, 1990*. The increasing importance given to the assessment phase of care management is shown by the titles and emphasis in these documents.

The guidance documents set out their own formulation of care management in seven stages; the first two stages are outside the circular process of care management:

- *publishing information* – to inform potential users of the service 'about the needs for which care agencies accept the responsibility to offer assistance, and the range of services currently available' (SSI/SWSG, 1991a, p. 11). This formulation limits the responsibility for providing information and turns the original American formulation of case-finding on its head: the aim is not to seek out cases so that they can be assessed and put in priority order but to define in advance what agencies will deal with. This may be an attempt to make clear at an early stage to the public that services will be limited, but it also meets the evidence, discussed above, that a clearly focused service will be more effective.
- *determining the level of assessment* – so that simple matters do not result in unnecessarily complex early work. Only complex and comprehensive assessment in the Practitioners' Guide's six levels of assessment (p. 42) would be undertaken by a professionally qualified care manager. The first three levels for limited services in low-risk cases would be undertaken by reception, administrative or basically qualified staff. Specialist assessments for particular services (for example, equipment for disabled people) might also be provided by specialist assessors, rather than requiring a full needs assessment.

After these two initial phases, care management is seen as a circular process which starts with stage 3:

- *assessing need*
- *care planning*
- *implementing the care plan*
- *monitoring* – which is concerned with checking how the plan is being delivered; and
- *reviewing* – which is a periodic review (and possible alteration) of the plan.

Reviewing then leads back to assessing need on the basis of the review.

The documents (for example, SSI/SWSG, 1991b, p. 14) define *need* as 'the requirements of individuals to enable them to achieve, maintain or restore an acceptable level of social independence or quality of life, as defined by the particular care agency or authority'.

This definition of need places the responsibility for determining acceptable quality of life wholly with the agency, rather than with the individual user of the service; client involvement is hollow: it is only relevant within the bounds of the agency's definition of the issue. Further evidence for this wholly imposed definition of needs is contained in the following paragraph, which indicates that need varies with changes in national legislation and local policy, the availability of resources and the patterns of local demand. In reality, the only acceptable needs according to this policy are those defined by legislation and the agency.

The Managers' Guide (SSI/SWSG, 1991b, pp. 72–7) also identifies a variety of possible models of care management, and some advantages and disadvantages of each. The two major divisions are between 'organisational' models (that is, those carried out within one agency) and 'inter-agency' models where the focus is on which agency takes the lead role. These interact: for example where one agency takes the lead role a variety of organisational models within that agency would be possible. Within these two divisions, definition of individuals', groups' or shared responsibilities need to be worked out.

One other feature of the Managers' Guide (pp. 81–105) is extensive guidance on inter-agency arrangements. This introduces the idea of the '*seamless service*' (p. 81) whereby, from the user's point of view, no joins in the service provided should be visible even if several agencies are involved. Three elements of policy will facilitate this: allocating lead responsibility to local authorities, having community care plans as a focus for joint planning and transferring social security residential care allowance finance to local authorities in 1993. Most attention is given to the NHS, but there is encouragement of liaison with other local authority departments such as housing and education, other statutory agencies such as social security and criminal justice agencies, the 'independent' (that is, private and voluntary) sector and the 'community' through community development work to increase resources provided informally and to increase public awareness.

Devolving 'some measure of financial authority' is also assumed in the Managers' Guide (pp. 36–7) to be necessary if responsibility is really to be devolved. The Audit Commission is invoked to argue that retaining budgets centrally prevents local authorities from meeting individual needs. However, Helen Smith (1992, p. 18) argues that delegating budgets means that responsibility for rationing decisions is diffused and could become idiosyncratic; an overview of rationing might well be lost and pressures would descend to and be hidden in lower levels of worker, where there is no influence on the policy decisions about resources, when it should be retained at a managerial level. Comparing this with the situation in the Kent project, the availability of resources there was absolute, provided that the requirements for achieving a package within the 'two-thirds of the cost of residential care' limit was met. Implementing devolved budgeting in a more restricted policy environment may not be viable, and since devolved budgeting is essential to cost-consciousness and to efficient operation, this problem may be a serious inhibition to implementing community care policy effectively.

As implementation of the Act approached, a variety of experiments and attempts at implementing care management were developed. In East Sussex, for example, projects were set up in primary health care setting such as health centres or GP practices (Harrison and Thistlethwaite, 1993). A relatively low number of clients was referred, partly due to hostility from professionals in the health and social services and uncertainty about what care management was. Few clients had full packages of care, and flexible budgets were little called upon, needs being met by the delivery of conventional services. This may have been because of lack of confidence among care managers, but there were also practical problems in ensuring accountability for expenditure and financial control. Similarly problems were experienced in Gloucestershire (Jays and Bilton, 1991). Although practice was needs-led, it was professionally-dominated. Care managers had difficulties because service users did not cope easily with the complex process of assessment and where there were conflicting views, it proved difficult to 'gain compliance' (p. 78). There was conflict with local user groups which had a philosophy of 'empowerment'. A Practice and Development Exchange Project for the DoH (Smale *et al.*, 1993) also identifies the importance of empowerment and the focus of assessment as crucial in making services responsive to the needs of service users. An *exchange* model of assessment where users and carers, as experts in their own needs, are facilitated to come to an assessment is preferred to a *questioning* model where an expert care manager interrogates each aspect of the care system and comes to a final decision, or a *procedural* model where the process is defined by rigid systems. This empowerment approach links more closely to the service brokerage approach to care management, whereas the government has preferred the Kent 'social care entrepreneurship' model.

Challis (1994), reviewing developments in the concepts of case management in the late 1980s and 1990s, argues that it will be an expensive failure unless there is clarity about target populations (the same point that Huxley makes, see Huxley, 1993), a reasonable degree of freedom for practitioners to develop responses, and clarity about care management's role in the wider system of care. Bland (1994), in a Scottish study, argues that care management is hard to implement because workers are not accustomed to working in an environment where they are encouraged to innovate and take risks, and there are fears about raising expectations which could not be met.

Introducing care management to community care: some conclusions

This section has explored in some detail the conversion of American conceptualisations of case management into care management in the post-Griffiths community care system. No doubt the concepts will develop and vary with local policies, but presumably DoH guidance will have considerable influence on the understanding of such a new concept.

I have argued throughout this section that, as the idea of case management has been converted from American concepts used in special projects, and particularly as official formulations have developed, the concept of care management has come to embody the central conflict in community care policy: between individualised, responsive care and the containment of costs. We saw this initially in the slightly different approaches of the Griffiths and Wagner reports. At the end of this process, need and the responsibilities of care management are defined always within the context of control of expenditure.

In practice assumptions, we have seen the development of an American concept which is primarily concerned with the co-ordination of services within in social work role, to a much stronger emphasis in British community care on 'assessment'. The Practitioners' Guidance (SSI/SWSG, 1991a) spends twenty-two pages on the two assessment stages of community care and twenty-eight pages on the remaining five stages. This emphasis probably reflects a long-standing social work bias towards defining assessment much more clearly than intervention, and the fact that these are early tasks to be undertaken in the process and so are more capable of generalised definition than highly variable intervention and monitoring approaches. I suggest, however, that it also reflects the concern for cost containment, since assessment is conceived of as a way of redirecting costs away from institutional care.

In organisation, the American concept of case management as being concerned with co-ordinating disparate resources has been maintained, but as a focus for the continuing concern of British governments since the Poor Law for developing co-ordination between the health and social services. This also has a covert cost-containment objective, since these two services are analogues, respectively, for 'more expensive' and 'cheaper'. At one time the political point might be made that central government was responsible for the health service and social security, and so shifting responsibility to the social services allowed responsibility to be hidden by blaming local authorities for failures, without accepting responsibility for appropriate funding. We have seen that devolved budgeting may widen responsibility further down the hierarchy among workers' individual decisions. However, this is made more complex by extensive delegation of responsibilities to local health trusts (and to take a distant example, schools). Localisation and delegation appears to be a general policy and management approach rather than something which is intended to hurt only local authorities. Local decision-making is also likely to restrain costs and increase the input of resources, because every budget-holder will attempt to stay within their budget, whereas holders of large budgets can have more of an overview and switch money around. Local people are also more likely to contribute small amounts of money which will add up to a large input, whereas holders of large budgets do not think such small-scale resource development activities are worthwhile.

It is a more helpful analysis to see care management, with its concern to delegate budgets and responsibilities locally, as another example of the government's management strategy of localising and individualising decisions in such a way that they are more responsive to demand. There are two objectives here. One is the simple assumption that centralised decision-making is slow and unresponsive to need: local and delegated decisions do away with bureaucracy. In a more complex way, it also means that operators of services (such as social workers and care managers) are forced to be more responsive to consumer demand than to political policy decisions, as I suggested when discussing consumerism in Chapter 1. The political assumption behind this may be that the clients will control the excesses of professional values (in the same way as the parents will restrain the educational establishment and the trade union members will restrain the political agitators). By privatising decisions (that is, by making then less open to public gaze and generalised analysis), we contribute to a Conservative political philosophy that the individual's decisions about themselves should be sovereign over collective policy strategies. The Conservative government may well hope that this will be so because many local authorities are managed by opposition parties who do not share this philosophy.

Allied to this, the emphasis on informal resources and others independent of public provision, has grown from the Kent project's demonstration that informal caring resources can be effective, positive and released by a small injection of public money. Griffiths's proposal of a wide range of providers, and the development by the government of the purchaser–provider split in this aspect of policy, as in others, emphasises the importance of co-ordination with private and voluntary providers. In a sense this was enforced on the social services by the growth of private providers of residential care in the 1980s: their involvement could not be ignored. Again, it is possible to discern a set of (Conservative) political assumptions lying behind the emphasis on this aspect of provision. A, possibly naïve, belief in the value of a 'family' and 'community' responding to needs that they see around them, reciprocating care in the daily round of life, is widespread. It is a Conservative philosophy that this was a reality, capable – where it is missing – of reconstruction. Hidden behind it is the assumption that women, particularly, should play this caring role in community and family life, and that doing so should be a priority for them over self-fulfilment in other directions. Again, we must note the cost-containment implications of promoting private sector investment in care activities, and the way in which informal care can contribute to relieving public costs.

Care management is the way in which that co-ordination of public with private and informal may be facilitated at the practical level. And social work, with its focus on the individual, the family, the community and its broad view of the links in the systems of relationships between these elements in society is the ideal basis for a form of practice which implements care management. Also, it has to be said, it is the ideal basis for implementing the Conservative philosophy which lies behind the way in which care management is being implemented in British community care. Social work practice is at the centre of the American and PSSRU conceptualisations of care management. As these have been been applied more broadly, a greater emphasis on multi-disciplinary work and user involvement has developed. The fact that co-ordination and devolved budgeting implies more management activity should not deny the importance of the crucial interpersonal skills of social workers. We can see this more clearly as, in the next three chapters, we look closely at the detail of care management practice in post-Griffiths community care.

Care management and social work

Having explored the conceptual and policy context of care management, then, we now turn to the role of social work within it. In Figure 1.1 (p. 2), the central role of care management was seen as containing slices of two much broader social work roles: the individualistic counselling/social work role and the community social work/social care planning role.

Care management involves the selection of individual cases which would benefit from intensive (and possibly multi-disciplinary) assessment, so that the best possible pattern of services appropriate to the individual may be devised and delivered. The philosophy is that the care manager starts from the needs of the client and moulds the package of services to those needs. Having devised the package of services, the care manager implements it through negotiations with a variety of agencies which might provide the services, creating a new and informal provision fitted specifically to the client. As the package is delivered, the care manager constantly monitors the services and ensures that they appear a 'seamless' service to the client. Periodically, the package is reviewed and any new factors in the assessment brought to bear to change the plan. Throughout, the client or user of the services is actively involved in making the decisions and contributing to planning, delivery, monitoring and review of the package. Within the American and Kent models, substantial importance is allocated to the counselling, therapeutic and interpersonal aspects of the social work role; this is rather downplayed in the largely managerial aspects of the DoH guidance; none the less, we have seen that it is essential if care management is to work well, and this is a strong focus of this book. We have seen that a more empowerment-oriented service-broker approach to care management with substantial elements of advocacy on the service user's behalf has been tried elsewhere, but has only limited application in the official guidance. Again, more of this aspect of the possibilities is emphasised in this book.

The assumption that care management will be better derives from the view that a single co-ordinator with an overview is better than a process of continual adaptation, and that in reality the services will respond to the co-ordinator. Another assumption might be that informal and community alternatives ought to make a larger contribution to care, and that a care manager can better facilitate this. Success here depends on the capacity of the care manager to develop such alternatives, integrate them with formal services and make them acceptable to clients. Early monitoring in 1993 suggested that in the first six months after implementation of care management policies, there was about 10 per cent diversion from residential care, through using more flexible packages (SSI/RHA, 1993). The Guidance also assumes that a care manager with responsibility for assessment and organising services will better represent the needs and interests of clients and users of services than people whose main focus is on providing services.

A lot is, therefore, being placed on the shoulders of care managers if post-Griffiths community care is to work in the way envisaged.

4

Assessment in Community Care

The aim of this chapter is to explore the role of assessment in community care, and to examine methods of assessment as part of care management. The first section identifies different assessment roles played by social workers in community care, and possible confusions between them. The second section looks at assessment as part of care management, according to the official guidance and other views. The first stage in the official guidance, that of publicising services and providing information to the public is reserved to Chapter 7, since it is at least partly a strategy for communicating with and empowering service users and their carers. The final sections explore multi-disciplinary assessments and involving clients and carers in assessment.

Assessment issues in community care

Assessment, because of its role in care management, is an important focus in post-Griffiths community care. It has its origins in at least four historical and sometimes confused meaning of 'assessment' within the social services, however. They are:

- *financial assessment* – of the amount a client pays towards the cost of a service
- *needs assessment* – of eligibility or suitability for a service
- *initial assessment* – at the point of entry to the social services
- *social work assessment* – as part of social work interventions which have therapeutic or other objectives.

How are these forms of assessment different from each other, and how have they become confused in community care?

Financial assessment has been a long-standing responsibility of social work and SSDs, and has a history stretching back at least to the Poor Law and the origins of professional social work in the 1890s. Most clients for community care services still need financial assessment for their contributions to the cost of care, and this proved to be one of the most difficult things to get right in the early stages (CRO, 1993). One official study (SSI/NHSME, 1993, p.16) argued that financial assessment gained a higher profile under the new arrangements. An extensive regularly updated guide is published giving details and containing relevant Statutory Instruments and DoH circulars (CRAG, 1992, 1993, 1994). A particularly difficulty in the early stages was the transitional payments made to continue to social security support given to people in residential homes prior to implementation of the Act. Subsequently, controversy has arisen about local authorities' discretion to ignore the value of a house owned by someone in residential care, which would usually contribute to the cost of care. Normally, the value of a house is ignored where a relative continues to live in it, but the local authority has discretion to ignore it in other circumstances too (CRAG, 1994, para 7.007). Social workers may have to get involved in arguing cases on behalf of clients or their relatives for disregarding the value of property.

Initial assessment is a basic function of SSDs. In intake work, people calling on the services of the department are quickly reviewed to gain a sketchy idea of their main presenting problems and the kinds of service that they might be considered for. This permits their case to be allocated to a suitable worker. In community care, this type of assessment is regarded as 'screening', since many applicants for service will not require care management, but simple referral for limited service. However, many SSDs, have not clearly distinguished this function from needs assessment. Instead, adult clients presenting potential long-term needs, particularly if they are presented as requiring assessment for private residential home care, may be assumed to require needs assessment. This tends to burden many cases with unnecessarily detailed assessment, and makes workers feel that the system has been made over-complicated and bureaucratic. The official guidance on assessment (SSI/SWSG, 1991a, p. 42) however, distinguishes different varieties of assessment, by differently qualified staff, depending on the client's circumstances.

Complex assessments by highly qualified workers should be a minority activity.

Needs assessment, as it should be for community care, develops the initial assessment and takes it forward. It is the function of care management. It requires a comprehensive analysis of need and the devising of a package of services. This simple statement is an inadequate reflection of reality: we need to make an excursion into conflicts about the origins and purposes of needs assessment.

One of the difficulties of introducing needs assessment into community care is its history as a form of practice in the pre-Griffiths system. Pre-Griffiths, clients or other agencies would request a service, or the worker would identify a problem which was interpreted as a request for a service. Assessment decided whether that service was appropriate, and would, perhaps, suggest other alternatives. In the pre-Griffiths system, a social worker would also have the responsibility (often not fully admitted, but this was the reality) of reducing the demand on services by suggesting alternatives which involved less commitment by the SSD by being less costly, or having a shorter waiting list.

This rationing or gatekeeping process is similar to post-Griffiths needs assessment, where the 'community care tariff' (see Chapter 5) gives professional respectability to cost containment. Even a genuine attempt to introduce choice into the options of an elderly person whose family wants her to enter residential care can be misinterpreted (or possibly accurately interpreted) by the family as an attempt to reduce costs. Budget management or awareness of cost as a part of care management dignifies cost containment as part of professional responsibility. It is also an important plank of the government's 'management approach' to the public services in general, as we saw in Chapters 1 and 2.

So, in practice, the worker's job is not *only* to carry out a full needs assessment and increase the client's options, but to limit the demands which may be made on the service. Obviously, these purposes might conflict. Suggesting community alternatives might have the later objective in mind, rather than the client's needs and wishes. Moreover, the awareness among workers and the public that the aim of the new service (which in general people support) is to increase the availability of community options means that the offer of community options might be made more acceptable both to workers and clients than it otherwise might be. Alternatively, reductions in

service or non-availability of some options can be made more pal-
atable to workers and clients than they otherwise might be.

The ethical approach to practice in this situation is to identify the
needs fully and recognise when these cannot be met, and this is the
principle which the Act appears to follow. However, by separating
needs assessment from the definition of the package of care, the
Griffiths reforms muddy the connection between assessment and
provision. The package of care is potentially infinitely variable and
negotiable. This enables client's preferences or worker's views about
appropriate service arising as part of needs assessment to be discounted, not only because they are not the best package of options
but also because they are too expensive.

This issue has been directly expressed in the debate over the 'Lam-
ing letter', the guidance issued to local authorities in the early stages
by the Chief Officer of the Social Service Inspectorate of the Department of Health. Paragraph 13 stages:

> An authority may take into account the resources available when
> deciding how to respond to an individual's assessment. However,
> once the authority has indicated that a service should be pro-
> vided to meet an individual's needs and the authority is under a
> legal obligation to provide it or arrange for its provision then the
> service must be provided. It will not be possible for an authority
> to use budgeting difficulties as a basis for refusing to provide the
> service.

This guidance raises serious questions, first, about the real commitment to user involvement in the system (see Chapter 7 below), secondly about the way cost implications might detract from decisions
about needs, and thirdly about the professional role of assessment –
that, is whether the professional decision about need and appropriate responses to it should and can always override financial considerations.

In the longer term, frequent needs assessment which could not,
for cost reasons, be met by packages of care would discredit the
whole system and lead to frustration and anger from clients or potential clients, their carers and workers. In political debate, it might
also be evidence that care management is being used primarily to
contain costs rather than develop a good community care system.
On the other hand, realistically, all possible needs cannot be met at

a reasonable cost to society, so compromises are always necessary. It might be argued that having a needs assessment made and identifying clients' wishes and workers' judgements at least makes more rational priority decisions possible. Also, a community focus encourages more people to come forward for assessment who would have been deterred from seeking help by the expectation that stigmatised residential care would have been the only option. At least then we can see whom we are rejecting rather than having a large area of hidden need.

From this diversion into issues about needs assessment, we return to the fourth kind of assessment identified above. A *social work assessment* is not just done once and then the whole of the work is based on it. Assessment of clients' needs and the work which is appropriate to meeting them is an integral and continuing part of social work interventions. It should be constantly reviewed and renewed as further information becomes available and deeper understanding of clients' needs and situations is achieved through the continuing work. The purchaser–provider split in community care might mean that this kind of assessment is inappropriate in care management, because it is not social work, but a way of creating a package of services. If social work is provided, it should be a service delivered by a provider.

However, we cannot make the distinction so clearly, for several reasons. First, the care management assessment is not a once-and-for-all event. It must be continually monitored and reviewed at regular intervals, and the principle of care management is that this should be done by the care manager as part of a continuing relationship which bears many similarities to social work carried out with therapeutic or other objectives. As a result, many departments do not clearly distinguish social workers offering social work services as providers, from care managers as purchasers. Frequently, therefore, care managers offer appropriate social work services themselves. Then, it is not easy to turn off the tap of assessment and turn on social work help; the two run into and constantly affect one another. An assessment helps clients understand and begin to work with their situation, and so begins to acquire social work objectives. Any form of social work, as I have suggested, requires constant reassessment as part of treatment, and this may well lead to changes in the care management assessment.

A social worker undertaking a care management role may, therefore, find several different elements of assessment included in the tasks that they must carry out. 'Screening' is a useful starting point for sorting this out in practice. If the SSD has not specific screening process, a care manager might reasonably identify clients who do not require a wide-ranging assessment and refer them simply for limited services. Where there is a screening system, but a client with minimal needs is identified, they can again be referred for limited service. Care managers can then concentrate on needs assessment, and they can consider the client's financial resources as part of developing a costed care plan. If social work service is required, it should have a separate plan and contract, with an element of costing associated with it, whoever is to provide it.

These confusions in care management assessment do not exhaust the different types of assessment which occur within community care. A simple system assumes a general assessment undertaken by a care manager, but more complex possibilities are envisaged by the DoH advice. For example, assessment might be carried out by a multi-disciplinary team; indeed Hughes (1993) argues that the need for comprehensiveness in community care assessments makes a multi-disciplinary assessment essential. A Scottish study (Taylor, C., 1993) found that multi-disciplinary assessment with older people was time-consuming, but produced effective assessments, and encouraged a more co-operative attitude to develop in the team. Better priority-setting and preparedness to express disagreement more openly would have helped decision-making. However, Royston and Rodrigues (1993), describing an integrated assessment scheme in East Sussex, argue that the care manager should be the focus of assessments from a variety of points of view. Such a process has a well-established history in individual programme planning, particularly with people with learning disabilities. Another alternative is that a general assessment may be followed by specialised assessments carried out by particular professional groups (for example, by speech therapists or physiotherapists) before they can offer their services effectively. It is important, therefore, to consider the relationship between the individuals carrying out the assessment work with clients, and other assessments or team decisions which will be required. In a Hounslow pilot assessment project (Hounslow SSD, 1992), most assessments for older people were in the DoH 'limited category, but it was felt that this was a misnomer, because clients' needs often required 'multiple' assessments from different services and these still had to be co-ordinated. Moreover, limited assessments were not always service-led; there was a move towards needs-led assessment in even fairly limited assessments. These points suggests that care management or careful social work may still be required, even where assessment are ostensibly quite simple.

The next section of this chapter, therefore, examines the assessment task in general. The final section looks at some of the issues which arise from the complexities of multi-disciplinary assessments.

Assessment in care management

Screening

Since it is the earliest pre-assessment stage, it is important to examine the possibilities offered by screening. A number of factors may screen clients out of the service, some of them not in the control of care managers or social workers.

- *Unawareness, stigma or poor publicity* This may mean that some people may not come forward, or may present their problems in ways which do not trigger a response from agencies. Similarly, looking at people who may be in institutions, the history of their behaviour or attitudes among professionals in, say, a long-stay hospital may mean that some people who might be assessed for discharge àre not put forward. Also, patients may not put themselves forward through fear of leaving the institution, when they might well benefit from the move if carefully prepared for it.
- *Pathways to the service may be convoluted* This may persuade potential clients that they service is not for them, or that they have particular needs which would not be met by the service (Payne, 1993b). Thus, advice that people are given by other agencies, and the expectations and advice given by people around them, conditions their view of the service and the possibilities it might offer. In one case, for example, Mrs Michaels had to consider the best arrangements for her son with learning disabilities, who was to leave school in two or three years time. A trusted teacher was jaundiced about the prospects of future employment for her son. Mrs Michaels, therefore, treated him

as fairly dependent around the home, and did not encourage the development of social skills and outside activities, which would have grown from his school work. When he left the education system, the multi-disciplinary assessment placed him in a social education centre with a relatively unskilled programme, and when Mrs Michaels became older, her son was placed in a large hostel, being thought unable to live independently. It was only at this stage in his care career that a fuller assessment of his capacities was undertaken, and a more optimistic programme developed. Some of these failings developed originally from the attitudes of a teacher fairly far removed from the care systems that made decisions about him.

- *Reception and intake* This is often done by poorly-prepared administrative staff who may be set in the ways of previous service patterns and may not have been fully trained in community care policy. Reception staff in social services agencies may see it as their job to protect workers from demands. The receptionist who says, in a kindly way, 'Oh no, we don't provide that sort of thing' is inconsistent with the idea that in care management workers will create a service which is appropriate, rather than offer only what is available. Training for reception staff may be an important aspect of service development.

- *Definition of initial problems* This may well be made in ways which minimise the complexity and just present a request for simple service. Mrs Venables, for example, is an elderly lady whose husband helped her with the practical work of the home until he died recently. Her daughter calls at the social services department asking for a home help for the shopping and housework. Mrs Venables may then receive a simple assessment just for this minimal service, and her emotional needs arising from recent bereavement and the importance of her existing level of disability and possible progression to more difficulties may not be picked up.

- *The population needs assessment* The department should have carried this out to identify the range of needs which services should provide for (Price Waterhouse DoH, 1993) and it may have led to some minority needs being ignored or discounted, or possible needs being missed in the department's systems and planning. For example, Mr Karim, from a small group of Punjabi residents in the area, called at a local area office, seeking help for his wife who was increasingly disabled with arthritis. However, contracts with a private home care service had not identified the need to provide staff with the language skills and knowledge of cultural requirements to give him confidence in the service which might be offered. Similarly, a day centre run by a relevant minority ethnic group was too far away in a nearby town; an extension to this town had not been thought necessary. These two failings left him very frustrated and he lost confidence in the ability of the service to provide useful help at all. This was disempowering for him and his wife because they could have no influence on what was provided for them to achieve a useful reaction to their needs.

Therefore, what an individual worker, an individual social services office or individual reception and intake staff do, and also the system that an agency sets up for screening and for planning community care policy generally, will have a minor effect on who comes forward for and receives help. An important element of screening will include, therefore, preparation of staff and creating forms for recording information which will record not only basic information but will ask for material which might identify problems requiring deeper exploration. Training or a form which alerts an intake worker to recent bereavement or stressed carers can be an important help in picking the right people to work with on a full needs assessment. However, at least one study has found that over-complex forms discourage flexibility and sharing with service users (Stalker, 1993).

Consistent with the policy of involving clients more fully in the process, workers might gain more complex and useful information in a cost-effective way (Raiff and Shore, 1993) from

- *a self-assessment form* which the client or carer prepares, so that a more considered view comes across; or
- *initial assessment in a group*, so that clients or carers can arrive at shared judgements about their referral: some might see that others have more important issues to face than themselves, others might be alerted to problems that they had not really perceived. This might be particularly useful in a dealing with groups of patients being discharged from hospital, but is easily adaptable to carers from the community referring relatives in need.

Such an approach may help to deal with some of the problems identified by Gomm *et al.* (1993) that assessment raises from a user perspective. They suggest that assessment is an action imposed upon someone from outside, and the idea of assessment is little understood by people outside caring agencies. Instead, they argue, we should talk about the tasks involved, such as deciding on needs, or arranging services. Their view fails to take account of the extent of self-assessment that is possible, and the way in which promoting participation in assessment can help people understand and make progress with problems themselves. However, the confusion in community care policy and official guidance of the idea of assessment as a helpful process (the traditional social work view) and as the basis for deciding on eligibility for services in short supply, feeds into the problems that Gomm *et al.* identify. However, early evidence (SSI/NHSME, 1993, p. 25) suggests that clients found complex assessments satisfactory, and carers felt pleased with the attention given to their needs.

We saw in Chapter 3 that there is some evidence that care management is more effective if it is used with clearly defined groups of people. One of the purposes of screening might therefore be to ensure that people with whom full assessments are made conform to the 'target population' that the care management service works with. This may be particularly important where we are concerned with rehabilitating groups of patients in hospital, where selecting appropriate people may strengthen the service considerably. However, in community teams with a wide potential population, screening may enable teams to identify clients suitable for assessment by particular specialists, or help general care managers to focus their initial assessment more clearly.

Information and its sources

Assessment is based on information, which may come from a variety of sources. Obviously, assessments of clients with different sorts of problems will require different kinds of information. However, there are a number of general formulations of the sorts of information required in social work assessments, and some of these are compared in Table 4.1.

The longest list is that of the SSI/SWSG guidance document, partly because it includes organisational requirements such as routine biographical details which are taken for granted in the more professionally oriented documents. Some categories which are more fully spelled out in one formulation are collapsed in others. However, a number of widely agreed categories do not appear under the major headings of the guidance. These include employment and activity (and for people with learning difficulties might also include training), recreation and leisure, education, and personal and social relationships (in their own right, as opposed to as part of a social support network).

From Table 4.1, it is possible to gain an overview of the kinds of information which might be included in an assessment, not only from a bureaucratic point of view but also including professional formulations.

Table 4.2 identifies areas of information which might be included in assessments where four or more formulations agree. These are further divided by the three dimensions of people's lives identified by Hughes (1993). The assessment of each of these relevant factors will need to include information not only on the present situation, but also on the potential for changes and what resources or possibilities might be available to achieve those changes. These two further aspects of the assessment are shown in the matrix in Table 4.2.

The sources of the information to be used in assessment are often taken for granted. In the case of the DoH guidance, this may be because of the emphasis on the users' and carers' definition of the issues as the main starting point. Other accounts offer a simple division of sources. For example, Taylor and Devine (1993, p. 11) identify three groups of sources:

- observation
- interviewing the client or clients
- other sources, both people and written records.

A more sophisticated formulation given by Moxley (1989, p. 28) covers:

- verbal descriptions of needs provided by the client
- collateral information about needs provided by social network members
- direct observation
- previous providers

Table 4.1 Information required in social work assessments

SSI/SWSG (1991a)	Moxley (1989)	Pilling (1991)	Hughes (1993)	Positive Publications (1993)	Payne (1993b)	Allen-Meares and Lane (1987)
General purpose	General purpose	Mentally ill people	Older people	Mentally ill people	Older people	General purpose
Biographical details						
Self-perceived needs			Attitude to self			
Self-care	Self-care	Self-care		Self-care		
Physical health	Health care		Health	Medical	Health and capacity	Physical state
Mental health	Mental health					
Use of medicines						
Abilities, attitudes lifestyles	Activities of daily living	Home management skills	Functioning			Behavioural, psychosocial environment
Race, culture					Oppression and abuse	
Personal history			Personal characteristics			
Carers' needs			Family			
Social network, support	Mutual care		Support network			
Care services	Professional care	Use of community facilities				

Housing	Housing, shelter		Environment	Financial	Housing, environment	Home, physical environment
Finance	Income					
Transport	Transport					
Risk: — hazards — health — behaviour		Anti-social behaviour				Behaviour
	Employment vocational			Employment	Employment	School, work
					Retirement activity	
	Social and personal relationships	Social skills and networks	Community relationships	Social	Personal, family and social relationships	Historic normative environment
	Recreation, leisure		Recreation activities		Leisure, social stimulation	
	Education				Education	
		Personal memory and orientation				
		Cognitive skills				Cognitive–affective

Table 4.2 *Information needs in assessment*

Present situation	Potential	Resources to achieve potential
A. The personal dimension		
Self-care, capacity to undertake required tasks		
Activities of daily living, ability to carry out		
Health and medical information, physical capacity for various activities		
Mental health, motivation		
Behaviour problems		
Financial problems and income		
B. Family dimension		
Family relationships and carers		
C. Community network dimension		
General social networks, and support and care needs provided from it		
Professional care services provided		
Housing and environment		
Employment and activity		
Recreation and leisure		
Education		

- review of records
- testing.

These indicate the importance of interviews with the clients, members of their households, people within their wider social networks and with previous or present service providers. Written records are also important, particularly so if the client is a patient in hospital or a long-standing client, where quite detailed information will be available. A problem with this sort of information is that previous opinion might blind us to the present possibilities.

These accounts also draw attention to two things which are sometimes underestimated. Direct observation of the client's skills and behaviour, perhaps in a new situation, may give a more realistic view of their capacities. Tests should also not be discounted. There is a variety of assessment possibilities particularly for people with learning disabilities, but also to assess mental states such as depression, and the degree of confusion and memory in an older person with Alzheimer's disease. If these are not available to the worker carrying out a care management assessment, the multi-disciplinary team may offer skills in using such options.

Another important aspect of assessment is to go beyond describing and the develop a more complex analysis of the network of problems that clients face (SSI/NHSME, 1993, p. 10).

Assessment aims

Carrying out an assessment is a process through which workers, clients and other participants move. The process has aims, some of which are administrative outcomes, some of which are care management and social work outcomes. The administrative outcomes concern the identification of:

● needs
● options for meeting those needs
● the views of clients and carers about the needs and options
● a reasoned judgement about the best way or ways of meeting those needs.

The DoH guidance (SSI/SWSG 1991a, p. 47) states that workers 'will have to make conscious efforts to treat the assessment of need as a separate exercise from consideration of service response.' Inevitably, though, exploring options and views about them begins to shade into deciding on what action to take about them, particularly when deciding on the 'best way' of meeting them. An early study (SSI/NHSME, 1993) showed that the organisational distinction between needs assessment and deciding on the services offered was not being maintained. However, it is important to maintain the distinction both for administrative and professional reasons, while recognising the value of connecting ideas about preferred provision which arise from the needs assessment with service planning.

Administratively, the local authority's duty to provide some response derives, as we have seen, from its assessment of need, so a clearly distinguished definition of those needs is important. Professionally, a clear view about needs and priorities offers a much firmer basis for explicit action and for helping clients and carers understand what it happening than a collapsing of thinking about need and action. The same thinking informs the practice of task-centred work, where it is important to explore and set priorities about problems before working out tasks which worker and client will carry out towards dealing with the problems (Doel and Marsh, 1992).

Hidden behind this apparently fairly simple set of aims for assessment are some complexities. We have seen how difficult the concept of need is. Saying that something is a 'need' rather than a 'want' gives it an imperative force (needs *should* rather than *might* be met), and placing this in the context of a semi-legal and administrative definition for the purposes of providing state resources strengthens that force still further. Deciding that a 'need' exists, therefore requires information to be collected and used as evidence to justify the imperative. Gordon (1993) shows that in collecting evidence for such purposes, local authorities have a legal duty to be 'fair'. This would require workers to get information from all the appropriate people, ensure that it is supported by evidence and make reasoned judgements based on the evidence, rather than being based on assumptions or rules of thumb.

The post-Griffiths community care model is inherently a *deficit* model of need. We can see this in the DoH guidance in statements like '[the] practitioner has to *define, as precisely as possible, the cause of any difficulty*' (SSI/SWSG, 1991a, p. 52, emphasis original). Other approaches are possible: for example, examining what would constitute a good quality of life and defining as needs aspects of life which would move towards better quality. Rather than seeing ourselves as running to keep up with escalating and unresolvable problems, it may be helpful for workers, clients and carers to see themselves as trying to identify ways of making positive progress in improving quality of life.

As well as administrative aims, care management assessment has some professional assessment purposes (identified in and adapted from Meyer, 1993) incorporated in it:

● engaging the client and carers in a process of assessment and personal and service development around their care needs;

- establishing a social environment in which observation and exploration of the client's circumstances can take place;
- advancing from and elaborating on the initial request or referral towards exploring and understanding issues and opportunities in the client's life;
- defining the nature of the 'case' and its boundaries, because workers do not deal with all aspects of a client's life – many things remain private and not the concern of the social services – and the boundaries of involvement and an understanding of why social services involvement is valid and ethical (this is what I mean by understanding the nature of the 'case') must be clear; and
- making judgements and inferences in an unbiased manner.

These two sets of administrative and professional aims in assessment must be borne in mind together when we approach situations requiring community care assessment.

The assessment process

The earliest stage of assessment is establishing the environment in which it is undertaken. The DoH guidance (SSI/SWSG, 1991a, p. 49) gives importance to choosing a setting in which the client will be comfortable and co-operation will be more possible. Raiff and Shore (1993, p. 29) recommend that work with clients should be 'in the ambient environment' the one that the client at present lives in. This helps the worker to observe the present situation and may make the client more comfortable, since it will be familiar. However, workers need to be alert to situations where the client may need to be assessed elsewhere because their home is too restrictive or a hospital ward makes them too dependent for the worker to be able to see their unused skills.

The worker also needs to establish a business-like but caring environment. Levin *et al.* (1989, pp. 297–8), for example, found in a study of services for confused elderly people that assessors were well-regarded if they were prompt; clear about who they were, who they worked for and why they were visiting; were sensitive and patient with the elderly people; listened to carers and were concerned about their problems; explained things clearly; understood the medical and psychological issues they were dealing with, and did not just accept a diagnosis, but went on to explore what the diagnosis meant for the elderly people and those helping them, and agreed a plan of action and carried it out efficiently.

Meyer (1993) divides the assessment process into five stages:

- *exploration and study* – information about the client's circum-stances, options, resources and action possibilities is gathered, selected and organised;
- *drawing inferences* – interpretations and judgements about the information, and, sometimes, explanations of what has happened are arrived at (these judgements then need to be checked with clients, carers and other sources of information and those who may have to take action; eventual action will be easier if the initial judgements on which a plan is based are agreed);
- *evaluation* – making a judgement about the strengths and weak-nesses in the clients' situation;
- *defining possible actions* – deciding what might be 'doable'; and
- *intervention and treatment planning* – this takes us into the next stage of care planning.

An important aspect of a community care assessment is not only the client, but also the social and care networks around them. Moxley (1989) suggests that it is necessary to look at ten sets of relation-ships

- people within the household (who may not always be relatives of the client)
- close relations, especially those living with or near the client
- relatives from the more extended family
- relationships made through work
- relationships within the neighbourhood
- informal relationships with people in the community such as shopkeepers or the milkman
- religious or other spiritual ties, and their meaning for the client
- contacts through clubs and social groups
- relationships with health, social service and other workers
- relationships formed through school, college, night-classes and so on.

Covering these areas in discussion with clients and their carers is likely to expose all the contacts in their lives. Moxley suggests that assessments might use the research techniques of asking about the amount of contact over various periods (say, in the last year) as a way of judging their importance. However, workers should be cautious with this: very close relationships may involve only occasional contacts, and supportive people may live at a considerable distance but offer emotional security because they exist and are prepared to help in an emergency. Seed (1990) argues that these should not be regarded as a 'group' since the members would not necessarily be in regular interaction with each other. He concentrates on the idea of 'meaningful contact', which concerns the importance of these contacts to the people involved. This is reflected in the strength of a network to the participants: a few really im-portant links may have greater strength than many unimportant ones. Seed points out that the links within networks vary over time and space, so that at some points during a period there may be more contacts than at others. Networks may also be more or less dense. More dense networks will have more of their members interacting together. The consequences of this sort of assessment for making and implementing care plans are considered in the next two chapters.

In looking at more formal services being used, Moxley (1989) also proposes a useful way of evaluating them, through the five As:

- *availability* – both whether they are present in the area and the extent to which the client and carer feels they are responsive to requests
- *adequacy* – whether they can only meet some of the needs or most of them
- *appropriateness* – for the client's particular needs
- *acceptability* – whether the form of service is acceptable to the client (for example, are meals provided at a day centre or delivered to the client's home suitable for their ethnic and cultural preferences)
- *accessibility* – are they near enough? can a disabled person enter the building?

In all of these it is important to be aware of the emotional element of each assessment – how clients and carers feel about them, and how they will work together with other services. If workers are assessing a wide range of services already involved with a client's situation, they will be in contact with a variety of services and their workers. If this is the case, a multi-disciplinary assessment may be more appropriate, and we now turn to the complexities of this type of assessment.

Multi-disciplinary assessment

There is no need for any aspect of care management to be multi-disciplinary. Care management, as a process, is intended to co-ordinate services provided by different agencies into a 'seamless' whole. These might be different services provided within the same disciplinary framework. Often, however, the services to be co-ordinated do come from different disciplinary bases, but because different disciplines provide services to the same person or group in parallel, this does not mean that the services are multi-disciplinary. (See Chapter 6 for a longer discussion of multi-disciplinary teamwork.)

This 'close-integration' form of multi-disciplinary work is, however, in opposition to some of the intentions of community care policy. DoH guidance (SSI/SWSG, 1991b, pp. 45–6) suggests that assessment should not be done for particular services, but by a range of staff covering many available services. The priority for staff is knowledge of a range of services and 'in-depth understanding of needs', rather than familiarity with particular services.

The guidance (SSI/SWSG, 1991b, pp. 50–60) offers a number of models for organising assessment both within an SSD and using inter-agency systems. There are fundamentally three forms.

- *Single assessor with consultation/involvement*   In this form, one professional assesses on behalf of the whole team, but consults others, and uses resources from other team members, some of whom may be seconded from other agencies, or part of formal co-operative links.
- *Single assessor with referral*   Here, one professional undertakes the main assessment, but refers on to specialists for assessments preparatory to taking up particular services for those who need specialised tests done. An example of such a process was the multi-disciplinary disability team in Westminster/Kensington and Chelsea (Pilling, 1992, pp. 132–78). This was outside the social

services and some views were held that effective inclusion of social services provision would be impossible. However, the fact that there was one worker provided continuity in contact with clients and services.

● *Team assessment* In this form, each member of a group of professionals who work together carries out different aspects of the assessment, which are then brought together, often in some form of case conference. This model has been particularly common in health care settings which are striving to become more involving of different disciplines. In primary health care settings in East Sussex (Harrison and Thistlethwaite, 1993, pp. 62–4) a modular assessment form was devised, so that different professionals could complete their aspects and be involved in the whole. A shared assessment document is a common means of co-ordination. In the Hounslow mental health project (Lawson, 1993), the care co-ordinator collected individual assessments (many on forms which are basically blank sheets and guidance notes), recorded the results of the meetings and worked out the plan based on the discussion. The All Wales Strategy for deinstitutionalising people with learning difficulties and more distant projects for this client group, developed the use of *Individual Programme Plans* (IPPs), where individual assessments were carried out and final decisions were made in a general meetings of the professionals, very often including carers and clients. This process has been developed widely in community mental handicap teams. Many of the Care in the Community Pilot projects (Knapp *et al.*, 1992) which were based on people with a variety of difficulties leaving hospitals also used multi-disciplinary processes for assessment.

One of the criticisms made of multi-disciplinary assessment is that it is time-consuming and involves substantial effort. Workers, clients and carers all build themselves up to a multi-disciplinary meeting, and after this time and effort find that the ideal plan cannot be provided due to lack of resources (Pilling, 1991; McGrath, 1991). The extent of effort required by multi-disciplinary approaches may, therefore, be even more counter-productive than the problem of lack of resources affecting assessments undertaken by a single assessor, unless there is some way forward to meeting the needs identified.

Involving the client in assessment

Community care policy makes the involvement of service users and their carers integral to the care management process. Gordon (1993) suggests that failure to involve the client and carer, and if desired to permit an advocate to speak on their behalf, may render the local authority liable to judicial review. This is, he argues, because of the importance given in the DoH guidance (SSI/SWSG 1991a) both to this and to the assessment as the precursor of the decision to award resources which requires the provisions of natural justice to be evident in the assessment processes.

Users and carers are traditionally the major source of information gained within social work assessments, so their involvement is not at issue. The crucial question is whether their involvement confers at least influence over decisions, and at most power or the right of choice? These issues are the main focus of Chapter 7; here I want simply to discuss aspects of the assessment process which may affect these issues.

Gomm *et al.*'s view (1993), discussed above, is that assessment is inherently an imposition of judgements by professionals from outside the client's position. One of the purpose of the post-Griffiths community care policy was, as we saw in Chapters 1 and 2, to interpose an assessment of need between the choice of entering residential care and the award of resources to do so through the social security system. We cannot, therefore, simply assume that involvement will mean influence.

Øvretveit (1993) provides a continuum of client involvement about decisions:

- no involvement
- informed or told
- consulted
- equal say, true veto, able to negotiate
- client-directed
- client or carer self-managed.

One of the problems with assessment, however, is that it is difficult in practice to identify when decisions are made. But we cannot delay involvement until the care planning stage, when the decisions may be directed by decisions made about need. Workers have to develop

Figure 4.1 *Simple explanatory assessment flowchart*

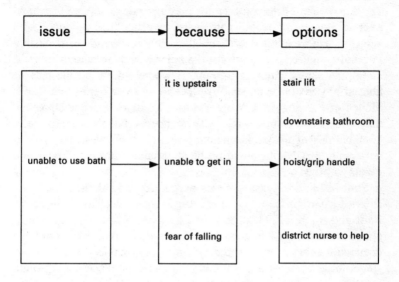

constant interchange with clients and carers about their thinking, including feeding back how the ideas they have expressed about their needs and wishes seem to the assessor. An important aspect of this will be simplifying the complexity of the matters discussed. It may be useful to devise simple written or visual formats, or perhaps simple flow-charts. Figure 4.1 gives an example of a visual flowchart explaining an issue. Three possible explanations are given in the second column of the fact that bathing has become an issue. For each explanation there is one or more option. A client can see easily how we move from the issue to explanations of the various options which would resolve the explanation. Providing a stair lift (an option to deal with the first explanation) would not help to deal with the fear of falling. Figure 4.1 also demonstrates the importance of raising emotional responses (fear of falling) as well as practical ones. Where there are deaf or hard of hearing people, visual formats are particularly important; with blind people, careful, logical accounts of the same information may be necessary to help them retain complex information.

An important set of emotional and practical issues which it would be easy to ignore in an assessment is the effect of oppression and discrimination against clients. In some cases, for example in dealing with people with learning disabilities, they may not be aware of the seriousness of this problem or may not raise it. There are, however, examples of people with learning disabilities in community settings being exploited or taunted by others around them. Such a possibility must be realistically appraised, and discussed with the client and carers. Another example is where elderly people may be abused physically or mentally by people in their family but this is hidden or unrecognised. Workers should look out for the signs and help clients and carers to raise their concerns. People from minority communities of all kinds, including ethnic minorities, may be experiencing disadvantage and problems arising from their status and others' attitudes.

Multi-disciplinary assessments may make it hard for clients and carers to participate in large meetings where decisions are made. Raiff and Shore (1993, p. 92), based on the American experience, are quite scathing about attempts to involve family members in large decision-making forums where they may be disconcerted by professional disagreements and not have enough experience of the forum to make a useful contribution. They propose moving beyond the issue of participation toward seeking to empower clients and carers to make knowledgeable choices. This involves giving them clear and adequate information, identifying possible options and the consequence of possible decisions.

Endword

In this chapter, we have explored how social work assessment and other forms of assessment in which social workers have been involved has become incorporated in the assessment phase in care management processes within community care. The separation of assessment from care planning, required by current policy, is both in process and in the conventional understanding of assessment an artificial division. In community care, assessment of needs will form the basis for moving on to make a care plan, and this process is the focus of the next chapter.

5

Care Planning

This chapter and the next are about care planning. In this chapter, the first section, on general issues concerning planning in social work and community care, identifies the 'tariff' implicit in community care policy which sets priorities within which planning decisions are made. Following sections about the practice of care planning focus first upon the role of social work within planning, then on identifying and working with existing resources which clients and carers already possess, including enabling, supporting and protecting clients and developing informal care resources. The final section covers the skills of negotiating the plan within the clients' and service networks, and also explores issues about informal care relevant to those networks. This chapter is, then, concerned with setting up the plan within, and developing, informal resources and networks. Chapter 6 covers the inclusion of formal resources and services in the package.

Care plans and the 'Community Care Tariff'

After assessment, care managers make care plans for their clients. The aim is to create a 'package' of care by selecting from existing services or developing new options which will meet the client's needs as they have been assessed. The care plan is at the centre of what will be provided for the client. Its creation will involve the client and may involve others around the client (for example, existing and potential carers and other service providers).

The plan will be about what is provided and also how it is provided. So, if the care manager decides that an elderly person should go into residential care, the kind of provision within residential care that would be suitable is identified, and how the client will be helped to make personal progress within their new setting. How such detailed planning is done may need to be negotiated, since the proprietor or manager of the home will make their assessment and develop their contribution. The client will also have a view, developing as experience of the new setting creates new views and opportunities. The care plan, therefore, will have several aspects:

● organising *initial* decisions about *resources* to meet the client's needs;
● early decisions about the kind of *help* offered to clients which will enable providers to make initial decisions about whether and how they will offer help; and
● the basis for *monitoring* and reassessment to identify changes in clients' needs, including changes in clients' views and changes wrought by providers as they take on aspects of provision.

Assumptions that are hidden in community care and agency policy form actual, but sometimes unacknowledged or unconsidered, objectives for the care manager in creating a plan. Thus, the DoH advises the care managers should:

● relate needs to available resources so that the assessment is practical rather than theoretical (SSI/SWSG, 1991a, p. 61)
● aim to promote clients' independence (p. 61)
● reconsider services rather than taking them 'off the shelf' (p. 62)
● discuss options with clients and carers, giving them choice and respecting their preferences (p. 62).

All these proposals seek to implement basic ideas in post-Griffiths policy. As well as this, post-Griffiths policy tends to assume a set of priorities about the preferences that care managers will have, which will colour the approach to planning. This is set out in diagrammatic form in Figure 5.1 to make, in effect, a *community care tariff*.

The main priority of the service is to maintain clients' independence, if necessary with informal care, and at this level, formal services are intended either to restore that independence, or maintain the informal care which enables it to continue. These services link to

Figure 5.1 *Priorities in service provision and development: the community care tariff*

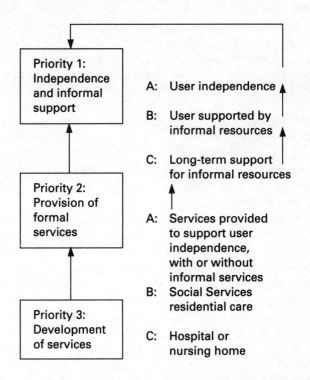

other formal services which seek to maintain a degree of independence. Beyond this, the priority (for reasons of cheapness) for residential care is to social services provision, with health provision coming last. The importance given to independence and informal provision implies that developing new provision in this area should have priority over developing formal provision. It is not essential to start at or seek to return clients to the 'independence' level; this may not be possible. None the less, generally, the assumption of the system (and probably the needs of most people) will mean that a worker will start planning at this point and seek to move as slowly as possible towards priority 2 options. If community care is to be genuinely preventative, involvement in difficulties at the early stages, as in the Kent Project (see Chapter 3) will use social work skills more effectively.

The 'tariff' may be overtaken by events. For example, a serious illness may deposit someone in hospital, leading to planning being made for discharge to a high level provision on the tariff. However, the assumption that someone coming from a high point in the tariff necessarily needs to work down the stages may not be valid. Someone may be in a hospital merely for one aspect of treatment. An elderly woman after a fall, for example, may need treatment for a broken leg and remobilisation when she is able to use the leg again. When that is dealt with, she may be able to return to a low point in the tariff. Another caution, though: the fall may indicate a degree of risk which means that more should be done, or different services provided from previously. This point will also apply when planning discharge for someone who is in care long-term. A complete reassessment of the point of the tariff at which they should be placed should be considered.

Part of the care planning process will include trying to strengthen the client's independence and developing informal care options at an early stage, therefore, and this aspect of implementing the plan will in many cases come before devising a package of care as such, although sometimes it will be the 'service' offered. This part of care management falls very much within the 'counselling/social wok' role among the three community care roles of social work identified in Figure 1.1. Looking at Figure 1.1 again as it appears in Figure 5.2, we can see how part of that role overlaps with the 'care management' role. Within that overlapping segment lies the initial process of strengthening the client's personal capacities – thus avoiding the need for more intensive services – or helping the client make better use of them. In the counselling/social work segment outside the care management circle would lie work done as a result of a decision to offer a longer-term social work aspect to the range of services planned. This would then become part of the package, offered as a provider function, even if it is carried out by the care manager.

Care planning: process and strategy

Since, as we have seen, the care plan is at the centre of providing community care over a period and through the phases mentioned above, it is obvious that care planning must be a process, rather

Figure 5.2 *The three community care roles of social work, showing counselling/social work roles in care management and as part of a community care package*

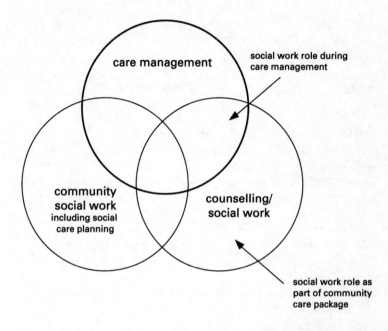

than a once-and-for-all activity performed at the beginning of a client's career in the community care services. Care planning is not a 'management' activity, in which a list of needs is matched to a list of services. It is, rather, a human interaction. Processes must be understood by seeing who is involved in them, how those people interact with one another and the outcomes of their activities together.

The *people* involved in care planning will always include

- a care manager (with possibly other care planning staff)
- a client
- representatives of services potentially involved

and may include

- actual or potential informal carers

- relatives, friends, neighbours and other people in the community with an interest in the client but who are not actual or potential informal carers
- one or more representatives of services affected by the client's circumstances (as opposed to those involved in providing services; for example, a GP may be affected, but will not usually provide a care-managed service).

A variety of *outcomes* to care planning is possible. The most obvious outcome is the actual care provided. Less obvious outcomes may include the feelings and responses of the people involved in providing and receiving the care; actual effects of the services on clients and the people around them; information which may affect the planning and management of services more widely; changes in the way agencies work; changes in the community which surrounds the client and how it responds to problems in its midst; and the information which provides feedback to the monitoring which will re-create the care plan in a new form as the client's situation develops.

In order to put this broad picture into action, it is useful for the care manager to have a sense of strategy; that is, where the care plan is coming from and its future overall direction. There are two aspects of where the plan comes from: the client's present situation and the policy and service context of the care management agency. These then move into the two aspects of planned future situation and the planned agency context of the care services provided. The dual perspectives of client situation and agency context can be classified as follows.

Client's situation

Understanding clients' situations must come from their own views. There may be uncertainty. For example, someone who sleeps at home may spend much of their day at a day centre in a hospital. The centre of their life, including their property and long-standing relationships, will usually be at home. It is easy to forget this, and focus on the care being provided in the day centre, when social relationships and experiences in the client's life at home may be much more important. As another example, Joel is an elderly man who is at present in hospital, having been admitted for treatment for a fracture after a fall at home. His friends and family are not able to visit very often, and his social life and treatment are all at the hospital, but he sees the hospital as only a temporary interlude; home is back at his house in the neighbourhood and with friends that he is familiar with.

Another more complex example is where the client lives in a group home. This may be their only home, and so be their 'home setting', but it is also a 'community setting' in the sense that it is provided as part of a caring arrangement.

Understanding the client's situation also requires identifying the client's networks. Networks are not necessarily 'support'. People's networks may reflect contacts which they have for many different reasons, and a contact for one purpose may need to be *converted* to a caring purpose: it cannot be assumed that the nature of the relationship can just be transferred. Joel, for example, is a member of the bowls club at the local institute; these are good friends, but he does not think that they might help him to get the shopping when he goes home from hospital. So Joel may not mention the bowls club to the care planner because it does not occur to him that its members might be relevant to caring for him. Also, he may be all too well aware of what the care planner might do, and he does not want to have all his networks recruited to caring purposes. In making care plans, we are looking for resources, but we must also recognise that boundaries do exist within clients' lives.

Another aspect of the client's situation is the condition or problem which leads to their needs being assessed. A clear definition of this should emerge from the assessment process. I place it last here to emphasise the importance of first evaluating clients' understandings of their own living arrangements and exploring networks in the process of creating a care plan.

Examining resources in the client's network

Workers are accustomed to exploring clients' networks, and usually agency procedures provide the facilities for this, through the forms that workers complete about cases. These generally include provision for identifying agencies involved with the client and the main relatives. It may be less conventional to seek information about other actual or potential informal carers, and the checklist of possible contacts in the previous chapter may help identify the possibilities.

Having gained the usual formal information, therefore, workers can usefully explore other people who might be involved in the client's life. Discussing a typical day or week may help to identify a pattern of behaviour which throws up links that may not have occurred to client or worker. It might be necessary to go back to the point at which a newly disabled person or someone in later life whose condition has been deteriorating was leading a relatively normal life. We should not ignore the mundane. For example, if Joel was a regular at the local public house, it might be more acceptable to arrange for someone to take him there for lunch than deliver meals on wheels or transport him to a day centre in the next town. On the other hand, if Jane has been a pillar of the Methodist chapel for fifty years, the local pub will get short shrift in favour of the village hall luncheon club.

Some people find listing contacts a lifeless way of identifying this information, and it can make it hard to see connections. Drawing family trees together with a client can be a useful way of understanding links, in an interesting way which involves the client actively. Similarly, a diagram of contacts with agencies and informal carers can be helpful, because it shows links visually; Figure 5.3 shows an example, based on the work of Seed (1990). He makes the point that networks are a pattern of links between points, and in the case of *social* networks, the links (as well as the people who are the 'points' on the network) have personal meaning to the people involved. Different kinds of networks relate to one another, so that relationships with particular people can be emotionally important because they are associated with particular places or activities. Various sophistications, such as showing physical distance by the length of line, may also help the visually minded and show some aspects of the client's situation which may otherwise go unconsidered.

Where clients suffer from problems due to disability, floor plans of their house or maps of their home area, showing where obstructions exist or what activities they undertake in which rooms, can also give a useful picture of ways in which work to overcome difficulties might be useful.

Agency context

Two fundamental points about agency context spring from community care policy:

Figure 5.3 *Simple network diagram*
(Based on Seed, 1990)

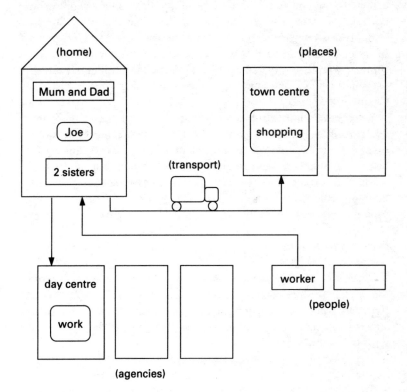

- the purchaser – provider split
- the co-ordination objective.

An integral part of post-Griffiths community care practice lies in the fact that purchasers of service, including care managers in the care management aspect of their role, must be separated from providers, even when employed by the same agency. Care managers may be an exception to this: as we have seen, they often provide an aspect of service, such as counselling or social work, themselves. However, management of most care services will be divided from the care manager, and may be part of a different agency. The general requirements of the service and the standards set for it will have been defined by a contract between the provider and the

purchasing part of the SSD or health authority. This may lead to
lack of flexibility in the kind of arrangements that a care manager
can make, or may limit the range of options for a client because
contracts are not available for particular arrangements. If this situation arises, one of the roles of care managers is negotiating ways
in which needs can be met within the requirements of the proposed
service. Another role will be feeding back the problems caused to
community care planning and purchasing parts of the SSD (see
Chapters 8 and 9).

Since community care is supposed to be 'seamless', care managers need to evaluate services to see whether such a high level of
co-ordination is possible. An important aspect of care planning may
be incorporating into the care package an element of support of social
work to form the 'glue' to hold the seams together. An alternative
is helping the user or carers to perform this co-ordinating function.
This has the advantage that it is within their control.

Care planning objectives

So far, in examining care planning strategy, we have been exploring where the care plan is 'coming from': the client's situation and
the agency context in which the plan is made. The second aspect of
strategy is where we are 'going to'; the objectives we hope to achieve
with the plan.

The DoH objective for care planning is

> To identify the most appropriate ways of achieving the objec-
> tives identified by the assessment of need and incorporate them
> into an individual care plan.   (SSI/SWSG, 1991a, p. 61)

This statement usefully emphasises the importance of starting from
the assessment of need. However, needs, once identified, do not
automatically lead to an objective and might be met in a variety of
ways. Some needs are more important than others, some may not
be relevant to community care services, and meeting all of anyone's needs that might be identified is clearly impossible. The constrained finances of community care might mean that even if meeting
an identified need were possible, the objective that it should be met
might not be attainable. Later in the relevant chapter, the DoH includes setting priorities, defining 'service requirements' and agree-

ing 'service objectives' as among the 'linked activities' involved in care planning (SSI/SWSG, 1991a, p. 61).

The statement also skates over the words 'incorporate', 'individual' and 'plan'. Let us start with 'plan'. A plan is an organised statement of action proposed for the future. Its basis is information gained about the client from the assessment, and also about possible resources. The DoH (SSI/SWSG, 1991, pp. 61–9) includes in care planning activities such things as exploring informal resources, reviewing existing services, costing the plan and finding out the client's means to contribute to the cost. Where there is a complex situation, or several connected clients, covering all these aspects in one plan may be difficult, and several linked plans may be more appropriate. Similarly, although plans are supposed to be for an individual, in some cases, a married couple may be involved, or several members of, say, a family with disabled members. Links between members of a family and their different needs should be clear and planned for. Similarly, clients' and carers' needs will interact; and need to be balanced appropriately (not necessarily equally). However, meeting a carer's needs must not interfere with the priority of meeting the needs of the identified client. In summary, the worker may have to consider a complex web of interacting needs, and design a complex plan to reflect this fact.

Remaining in or moving into the community

An important distinction in care planning must be made between those clients who are moving from an institution, particularly if they have had a long stay, and those where the aim is to prevent admission or provide extra care to assist people in the community. One difference may lie in their social and practical skill and psychological strength. People who have had long stays in hospital may be able to do less for themselves, may find it less easy to form relationships and may start from a position of greater disillusion than people who have lived independently. On the other hand, people in the community may be on a downward spiral when help is sought and so they may be unconfident of their abilities and strengths, whereas people in a hospital being made ready for discharge may be optimistic as well as fearful. In some cases, bereavement may blunt their capacity and motivation.

Another important difference between these two groups is that care planning for discharge allows a comprehensive plan to be made in the beginning, and preparation, training and facilities developed over a period, whereas care planning for someone already in the community places the worker in the middle of a situation and requires immediate and very often partial action. This may compromise future possibilities, so one of the important things to do when approaching care planning in the community is to take early and emergency actions so as to leave options open.

The process of care planning

Care planning starts with the people involved and moves towards the general objectives and priorities identified above. Social work skills throughout the process will engage the client and others involved in relationships which will enable them to participate in the process. Raiff and Shore (1993) emphasise the need to pay attention to that relationship aspect at all times, and not to attempt planning unless a satisfactory relationship exists. The *interaction* between the people involved always starts from the client's present situation and evolves through:

- an introductory phase in which the care manager enters a relationship with the client and the present situation;
- an assessment phase (see Chapter 4);
- a formulation phase, in which the care plan is established in a basic form;
- an agreement phase in which commitment to the plan is achieved among those who must do so in order that it can be implemented, including the client and close personal carers;
- an implementation phase in which the plan is put into action; and
- an operation phase in which the care arrangements made work within the client's life (see Chapter 6).

Within the formulation phase Moxley (1989) proposes the importance of identifying the particular areas of need that will be addressed in the plan (for example, housing, particular disabilities) and then to create specific goals to achieve. He proposes that these should be defined in terms which can be readily evaluated and include defined tasks for identified people and time limits within which particular tasks should be performed. To look at an example of this, Mrs Finnery is an elderly lady living alone, previously cared for by a middle-aged daughter who has suffered a life-threatening illness, and is no longer able to offer personal care. One issue is finance, and attendance allowance (for people aged over 65, disability living allowance does not apply – Poynter and Martin, 1994) needs to be explored. An assessment of Mrs Finnery's safety, feelings about her situation and preferences for services needs to be established. Her daughter is prepared to approach two long-established neighbours and friends for help, and the worker agrees to begin negotiations with the nursing service and refer for assessment for home care, to investigate day centre placements, night-sitting and (inessential, but good for morale) a period away on holiday. Mrs Finnery, in the meantime, has discovered that, moving carefully, she can manage to prepare light meals herself. Each takes on a role and agrees to report back in a meeting in a fortnight's time. While planning is going on, therefore, some progress can be made, at least on an interim basis, everyone is involved and nobody has to sit back and wait.

Raiff and Shore (1933, p. 36) usefully recommend planning and implementing the plan in parts, so that clients or helpers are not overwhelmed by the extent or complexity of demands upon them. They also emphasise (pp. 42–3) the importance of five standards of planning:

- logical development from assessment, so that clients and carers can see and be committed to the steps
- start with long-term goals which lead to developing short-term goals
- make short-term goals realistic and attainable in the view of clients, carers and workers
- take goals one by one and set a clear specification of action, outcomes and who does what within which timescale
- be brisk and decisive, thorough and involving.

Many of these ideas relate directly to task-centred social work, a popular model of social work practice, widely used in the UK (Doel and Marsh, 1992).

Skills in care planning – making best use of clients' resources

All clients being assessed will have their own resources to contribute to the situation. It is important not to neglect these and to develop their use so that they make a bigger contribution to clients' lives. They will include:

● physical resources, such as a house or flat, furniture, and household goods, transport
● emotional resources, such as perseverance, optimism, caution
● skill resources.

A helpful way of thinking about possibilities of action with a client's own resources is to consider:

● *making space* for the client to use resources which they cannot bring into play (for example, providing aids and adaptations to the house of a disabled man so that he can carry out cooking and personal tasks, rather than relying on his mother);
● *giving direction* to resources which are not proving useful at present (for example, organising a neighbour to call at a time when someone is at risk because of a gap in the timetable of carers visiting); and
● *focusing* the client's activities more helpfully (for example, encouraging the client to concentrate on personal care and domestic tasks, leaving the home help to undertake more complex and risky tasks)   (Payne, 1986a).

The social work skills relevant to improving the use of clients' own resources are those of enabling, supporting and protecting.

Enabling

Enabling aims to put people in the position to use resources that they already possess, but which circumstances prevent them from using. Possible strategies include the following.

● *Extension* – identifying skills or resources which the client is already using and improving their ability to use them more widely. Mr Talbot, for example, is a man with learning disabilities, liv-

ing with a group of three others. He is a pleasant, friendly man
at the day centre, but like the others does not use local community facilities. Teaching him skills in making social contacts
and behaving appropriately might help him to act as a leader in
picking up some simple social activities in the neighbourhood.

- *Stimulation* – encouraging new ideas and positive feelings about
  developing new activities or skills. Mr Talbot will need encouraging to feel that he will be able to use his existing social skills
  more widely, and not be put off by the lethargy of some of the
  people he lives with.
- *Accommodation* – changing the environment around the client
  so that they are able to use skills that have previously been
  restricted. Arrangements could be made with some friendly neighbours to invite Mr Talbot and then his co-residents for simple
  social events. Later, helping them financially and practically to
  use local evening classes, if necessary encouraging the adult
  education centre to develop suitable provision, might facilitate
  further development.
- *Transfer* – helping a client to see that skills he or she already
  has can be used in different situations.
- *Approximation* – helping a client to make progress in the desired direction by easy stages. For example, an elderly woman
  who has had a fall in the street was so frightened by the experience that she confined herself to her home. The important approach was to deal with her fear, and physiotherapy was offered
  to help her feel more confident in her muscles and movement.
  Then she was given a programme of movement around the house;
  once confidence was developed, she was able to try going into
  the front garden, and a relative bought a suitable chair for her
  to be able to sit out. This enabled her to talk to one or two
  passers-by. Eventually, she walked to a nearby shop, and later
  to other local shops.
- *Side-stepping* – avoiding an obstacle by helping to find another
  way round.

Much of the worker's activity in enabling will be concerned with
explaining, educating and informing clients and the people around
them. Useful areas to consider are people's understanding of the
behaviour and circumstances they are involved in, their understanding of the services being offered and of their own role.

Another area to consider is trying to be specific about the problems, behaviour or options people are considering. The daughter of Mrs Knowles, a frail elderly woman, for example, was appalled at the suggestion that her mother should remain at home rather than going into residential care, and reacted very aggressively. The worker sat down with her and defined exactly what the risks were that she was concerned about – for example, falling when there was nobody present, poor nutrition and in particular the possible restriction on the daughter's work opportunities if she had to take time off to care for her mother. Against each of these difficulties, the worker was able to construct a day or domiciliary care option which met the problem; occasional substitute care through a night and weekend sitter scheme and the availability of respite care also helped her to accept that this was a valid set of options for her mother, which also maintained her own independence and allowed her to make a, limited, contribution which she felt she could manage. Workers should, as in this example, help people tell them about problems which they may feel are 'selfish', but in fact reflect very real needs in their own lives. Similarly, they need to explore views which are wider than those of the people apparently involved. Mrs Knowles's now dead husband thought that daughters should always care for elderly parents and this had caused difficulty in the household when the daughter was in her teens, and she feared that her mother would hold this view and view her badly if she did not provide care. Her own husband's anxiety about disruption of their income was also a factor where anxieties had to be allayed.

Other situations in which it is useful to be specific is where there are complaints of difficult behaviour. It is necessary to find out precisely what behaviour is presenting the problems, and when it occurs. From the patterns that can be identified, workers can often see situations which set off difficult behaviour. By avoiding the triggers, the behaviour problems can also be helped to disappear.

Some people in social work use the words 'enabling' and 'empowerment' interchangeably. I do not think this is right. We have been discussing here responses to a particular situation, which may enable clients to deal with it, in their own way and according to their own priorities, but the worker is very clearly operating as a professional responsible for the outcome. The experience of taking part in this may be empowering for the client, in the sense that it helps them overcome obstacles to action and gain control over aspects of their lives which were previously out of control. But enabling in a particular instance may not be more widely empowering. If workers can operate in ways which achieve this, it helps clients gain more power over their lives, and is consequently a useful aspect of enabling.

Support

Social workers often talk about providing support to clients and carers, but are just as often criticised for using it because:

- it implies merely keeping still, rather than improving the situation, or developing the client's power over their lives;
- it is hard to define clearly what you are doing when you are providing support, and so it is hard to explain this to clients – this means that they cannot participate so readily, and, again, lose power over their lives;
- related to this, it is hard to have clear objectives.

Some of the criticisms derive from an assumption that social work should always aim at therapeutic progress instead of preventing deterioration in existing situations or making people feel safe and happy where immediate progress is not possible. Safety and happiness are worthwhile achievements. Since community care is about long-term work, support may well have useful aspects, provided workers try to be clear about what they aim to achieve. The following discussion tries to analyse what may be involved.

Sometimes support comes from the client's knowing that the worker is involved, and depends on *how* the worker relates to a client, rather than what is done. This is integral to the approach of social work to dealing with members of the public, and falls into the category of supportive activities which Compton (1989, p. 568) labels 'use of relationship'.

Compton identifies another aspect as 'use of resources'. I have previously argued (Payne, 1986a, pp. 37–41) that this form of support arises where social work activities 'take over temporarily certain aspects of the client's living'. Here we are moving from within the care management role towards organising services as part of a package. The social work element of developing packages of care may well comprise the supportive element. The support is the glue which holds the construction together, and needs to be a planned part of the package.

Generally there are three parts of support, as an aspect of a care package:

● *availability* – where the worker helps the client feel secure in the knowledge that there will be a response if necessary;
● *substitution* – where aspects of the client's life are taken over by the services, in order to help the client operate more independently in other areas; and
● *involvement* in an important change – so that the client, relying on the relationship aspect of support, can gain experience of and confidence in functioning in a new way, before managing on their own.

For example, Mr and Mrs Walker were an elderly couple living together. Both were increasingly frail, and a crisis arose when Mrs Walker was to go into hospital for an operation. This had been planned, however, and the general practitioner had referred the couple for help. The worker formed a relationship with both of them, and since the admission date was uncertain, planned various options to provide increasing care for Mr Walker, if problems arose. The worker offered office and home telephone numbers, so that they could contact her in any emergency, thus demonstrating her availability. Availability is a psychological part of the relationship as well as being a practical one – giving a home phone number rather exceptionally helped the couple to feel that here was someone who was prepared to put themselves out for them and respond when they wanted, and not only in office hours. When contacted a week later about another difficulty, her immediate visit gave the couple a feeling of confidence. We see here both relationship and availability aspects of support.

When the admission came, Mr Walker was provided with a home help, who carried out tasks which he was too immobile to undertake. This is an example of substitution. The worker kept in touch with the home help and both clients, and also arranged for Mr Walker to make some visits to the local town with a volunteer; an 'involvement' aspect of support. Finally, when Mrs Walker came home, home help service was increased, the worker negotiated a phased withdrawal of help, and also arranged meals on wheels and some further outings for both old people. Here, she actually increased support at the time of change, even though apparently, the problem was at an end when Mrs Walker returned home. It is often important to identify the difference between a change which resolves a situation (and can lead to reducing support) and change which increases difficulties because of the stress involved in change itself (which can justify increasing support to help cope with the change). The worker provided both involvement and substitution, and by being active at the time of the return home, she also demonstrated her availability again. By negotiating over arrangements, 'psychological' availability – a preparedness to get involved and an openness to being influenced – was made clear to the couple again.

Protection

Protection extends and builds on support. Many people under pressure in the community, either because they have been discharged from a more secure environment in a hospital or because increasing pressures are affecting them, need protection to preserve their psychological and physical strength and to prevent damage. Sometimes agencies take the view that it is important to avoid all risk. Clearly this is not possible, and the best approach is to try to be clear where risks are and try to combat them.

Organising protection requires, first, an assessment of risk. Brearley (1982) argues that all situations involve some risk, so we must look at how serious any particular set of circumstances is. Risk has two elements: the chance that something will happen and the seriousness of the consequences if it does. A hazard is some factor which could produce an undesirable outcome and a danger is the possible outcome. There are hazards which might predispose people to risk: for example an elderly person might be increasingly frail, or someone with learning difficulties might be unable to understand or perceive potential dangers. Other hazards exist in the situation and are likely to make it more risky, for example if the carer of an elderly person falls ill, it is more likely that things will go wrong.

If we look carefully at any situation, then, we can try to see where the hazards are and where the dangers are likely to be. Various options for protection might involve:

● *removing hazards* – such as unsafe furniture, or by substituting for a carer who is no longer able to care;
● *avoidance* – by moving someone to a new room in the house,

or avoiding the need for them to go upstairs, or advising someone who feels threatened by local youths about safety precau-
tions;
● *reducing or removing triggers* – by preventing events arising
that lead to potential hazards, for example if a man living alone
drinks a lot and is at risk of falling, it might help to try to
reduce his drinking or encourage him to drink in safe environments or where other people can keep an eye on him.

Such strategies are most effective when the client can be involved
in the preventive measures. This helps to alert them to problems
and to identify other difficulties which might be more apparent to
them than to a worker. It also engages them in actively seeking to
avoid the difficulties themselves; co-operation will be essential where
an element of behaviour change is required.

Informal carers

An important element of any care plan is the people within the
client's network who already provide care, or who might do so in
the future. As well as considering enabling, support and protection
for the client, workers will consider the role of informal carers in
the care plan. We have seen already that community care policy
gives high priority to their involvement, because of:

● greater awareness of informal carers' importance and contribution;
● awareness of stresses on carers and their needs for support: they
may become less efficient at work, experience pressure on family finances and themselves suffer physical and mental ill-health
(Perring, *et al.*, 1990; Parker and Lawton, 1994). However, most
care is essentially practical (about 72 per cent), rather than physical
and personal care (about 29 per cent) (Parker and Lawton, 1994);
● the inability of official services to meet all needs;
● clients' preference for informal care;
● government ideology and its stress on the family as the basis of
social life, and as a preferred basis for social provision.

Before simply accepting the community care tariff which gives priority to developing informal care, however, it is important to explore the nature of it, and what it can and cannot offer to the community care system. Such an exploration falls into three questions:

- What is informal care?
- Can it be made available?
- How may it be supported?

What is informal care?

Informal care means care provided to individuals by people in contact with them through links which have not been created in order to provide that care. Usually, informal care is provided by relatives, friends and neighbours of the individuals cared for, through links which come about through kinship, common interests or the fact that the people involved live close to one another or work or have worked together. Wenger (1994) argues that there are a variety of different types of network, which should be assessed. These are based on:

- the proximity of close kin
- the proportions of family, friends and neighbours involved
- the amount of interaction between people (in the case of her studies, older people) and their networks.

She identifies five types of network, which care managers might find it useful to consider:

- family-dependent support networks – with their main focus on local kin;
- locally integrated support networks where there are close relationships with local family, friends and neighbours;
- local self-contained support networks where there are infrequent and rather distant relationships with local kin and informal networks;
- wider community-focused support networks where there are active relationships with distant relatives, but relatively few local contacts; and
- private restricted support networks where there are no local kin and minimal contact with others in the local community.

Different types of network offer different opportunities for developing informal care and call for different approaches from the care manager. Wenger (1994) proposes an instrument for assessing the type of network surrounding an older person.

To understand informal care, we must look in turn at each of the three types of carer and some of the issues which arise with them.

What are the differences between relatives, friends and neighbours? Relatives are forced on us, although we can reject the relationship. Friends are chosen, and a level of intimacy in which we give up varying degrees of privacy is an essential element of friendship. Neighbours are unchosen, except if we can choose where we live and take the neighbours into account in making the choice. There is generally less investment in relationships with neighbours, but they may grow into friends (Bulmer, 1986, pp. 96–9).

Relatives often provide care for each other alongside other aspects of their relationships which derive from their kinship. The importance of their relationship may come from the length of a relationship based on kinship and shared experiences, formally acknowledged ties, such as those initiated by marriage vows, the fact of living together or near each other, and personal and emotional similarities which derive from shared genetic characteristics. Social expectations about the role which relatives will play in the lives of their kin are a particularly important feature of caring roles among relatives.

For many people, kinship is an important part of their lives. Willmott (1986) identifies four types of kinship networks:

- *local extended families* – where involvement is with a large number of relatives and they all live fairly close together; this is typical of working class families in stable communities;
- *dispersed extended families* – where a large number of relatives is involved, but they live well apart and contact by telephone and car on a regular basis is important, and is associated with regular practical help;
- *dispersed kinship networks* – where contact with the nuclear family and grandparents is maintained mainly by phone and letter, with occasional long-distance visits, and crisis help;
- *residual kinship networks* – where there is some contact, but relatives are only rarely seen.

Relatives and especially spouses provide the bulk of care for elderly and infirm people and others (Bulmer, 1987). Visiting to provide social contact, practical help with shopping and cleaning, and 'tending' which helps with more intimate personal tasks, such as bathing and feeding, are all carried out by relatives in many instances.

Feminist perspectives have been crucial in identifying the 'gendered' nature of family caring, since it is the female members of families upon whom the burden of caring often falls because of assumptions about the role of women in society and in relationships, particularly within family relationships (Graham, 1993). Moreover, it is assumed that it is 'natural' for women to provide care in family relationships, and part of their emotional and personal nature, and that they do so without payment, it may be assumed that they will do so in other situations, as neighbours or friends, and that they will take on caring roles in formal services, but will accept honoraria or low payment for taking on such work. Cohen and Fisher (1988) found in a survey of mentally ill clients of social workers that the workers tended to focus on the client and ignore the needs of carers, especially if they were women.

Men in this situation, it is argued, are more likely to receive formal help in caring. Parker and Lawton (1994), however, found that they tended only to get more domestic help, the level of other services being similar. The feminist analysis has led writers such as Dalley (1988) to propose that collective forms of care are more appropriate than the individualism and 'familism' that we have seen is an integral part of post-Griffiths community care policy. However, this has been criticised from the perspective of the 'disabled living movement' by Morris (1999), who argues that for people who seek complete independence, collective solutions may mean residential home options or excessive control of their lives by formal services. It is also important not to misconstrue the 'gendered' nature of caring. Arber and Gilbert (1989) analysed the role of men carers and found that one-third of carers who live with the person being cared for are men, usually with a strong personal bond. Once the level of disability of the person being cared for is taken into account, these men received much the same level of formal help as women. Parker and Lawton (1994) found that they were less likely to be calling on medical advice, but otherwise use of services by people being cared for by men was similar to those used by people being cared for by women. Women caring for other women received fewest services. The type of household is the crucial variable; formal help is less when there are younger members of the household. The major imposition on women is where married daughters are caring for elderly relatives, since although they are young, compared with an elderly spouse, they have other caring responsibilities, such as caring for their children, which are not considered in allocating formal help.

The most important question which needs to be asked about informal care from relatives is: why do they (rather than anyone else) feel the responsibility or obligation to care? Post-Griffiths policy tends to assume that this is natural, based as it is on the assumption that the family should be the basis of social life. Finch (1989) argues that this is not so, and that a series of social 'guidelines' are a more appropriate way of understanding the complex set of expectations and excusing conditions around which family responsibilities are negotiated. A subsequent study (Finch and Mason, 1993) shows how people balance responsibilities and commitment to different members of their families, how who does what may be negotiated over time and a pattern emerge which is thought right for that set of relationships, and how commitment to another builds up over time. Important features are that the person in need must be 'deserving' in the sense of not being to blame for their predicament, where the commitment and effort required is fairly limited and where parents and children are involved, although responsibilities of children to care for their elderly relatives is less well-defined than that of parents to provide for children.

One area of concern is the needs of carers from minority ethnic communities. A comprehensive survey of the research by Atkin and Rollings (1993) showed that because of demographic factors, needs for care services among minority ethnic communities are likely to increase during the 1990s. There is a low level of knowledge and use of services at present, irrespective of age and disability, although black minorities are interested in using services. Information materials and channels directed to their needs will be crucial developments. Norman (1985) described the position of older people in minority ethnic communities as one of 'triple jeopardy', since they are at risk because they are old, because of the problems and social difficulties which often afflict older people and also because services are not organised to provide for their special needs as people from minority ethnic communities. Jackson and Field's 1989 study of voluntary sector services shows that some Asian people did not translate knowledge of services into use, because they were unsuitable for particular cultural needs, because of discrimination and because of fear of discrimination. They found some evidence of a preference among some Asian people for the use of family support. Because this preference exists, it is important not to assume that the support will be available. There are some indications that professionals may be making unwitting discriminatory decisions in considering needs. Since need assessment is basic to community care, such a failing would have extreme adverse effects. However, Atkin and Rollings (1993) could find little evidence of concerned implementation of policy within statutory services to respond to this issue. Well-known strategies such as employment of staff from black and ethnic minorities, using interpreters and ethnic monitoring have had little impact on provision.

The worker has to consider these issues when dealing with family care. It is important to be aware of the possibility of making impositions on women as carers, because of social assumptions about their role, or about minority ethnic communities because of some preference for family care. In particular, workers need to consider their other caring responsibilities. For example, Renee has two sons, both at crucial stages of schooling, when her father, who lives alone nearby suffers from a stroke, and returning home after treatment, needs regular visiting, meals to be provided and some physical care. Planning her role in relation to formal services should take into account her sons' needs and the space she must have available to provide adequately for them. Finch and Mason's work also demonstrates how important it is to see that the role which she might play might be affected by the history of the relationship with her father and how members of her family see caring roles as part of their relationships; perhaps such roles are assumed, perhaps they are abhorred.

Friendship is the second form of informal care. Friendship indicates a personal bond which does not come from a sexual relationship or from family ties. Willmott (1987) defined friendship according to the amount of contact in social networks, and also according to what kinds of help would be offered by friends to each other, and found that this mixture of factors provided a realistic basis for asking people about their friends. He found that people identified the main characteristics of friendship as trust, respect for privacy, being prepared to be confidantes and being pleasurable social companions.

Richardson and Ritchie (1989) propose that friendship offers intimacy, company and practical help. We gain friends at different stages in our lives, such as school, college, work and through shared interests and needs; for example, when children are young, people make friends with other young parents. Class and social context, gender and stage of life are the major influences on how we make friends and who with (Willmott, 1987, p. 5). Most friendships have an important element of reciprocity and exchange. Each party to a friendship or group of friends offers something to the others and takes support in return. Allan (1983) argues that this does not contribute well to caring of a more personal kind, because the element of exchange is lost.

As a result, most studies show that friends are not a major source of social care (Willmott, 1986). They may, however, provide particular kinds of support. In particular, the social contact and companionship may be a useful emotional benefit to people with care needs, and the aspect of private, confidential discussion is also a beneficial element of stress reduction. This may be particularly so for people with serious difficulties who have not had opportunities to develop friendships. Richardson and Ritchie (1989) studied people with learning difficulties. Outside work or formal care provision such as day care, they had few social contacts, partly because they had a limited social circle. These people experienced a lack of intimacy and companionship in their lives. Richardson and Ritchie suggest that efforts should be made to offer this, by widening their social circles and providing opportunities in which friendships might arise. Sometimes, formal befriending schemes can help, but these inhibit the sense of choice which should go with friendship.

Workers need to be aware of the benefits of friendship for all groups of their clients, and try to find ways of increasing friendship networks or re-establishing links that have dried up. This is important for clients' social and emotional well-being, and may enable them to manage difficult lives more effectively. However, many friendships will not be appropriately converted into providing personal care.

Much the same might be said of help from *neigbours*, people who live near one another. Abrams (Bulmer, 1986, p. 21) defines 'neighbourhood' as a defined locality inhabited by neighbours, 'neighbouring' as the pattern of interaction within the neighbourhood and 'neighbourliness' as a positive and committed relationship between neighbours.

The reason for interest in care from this source links to political assumptions and social myths about 'community' in the same way that care by relatives links to similar assumptions and myths about 'family'. The post-Griffiths community care tariff, discussed above, assumes that neighbours will and should care for each other. Abrams (Bulmer, 1986, pp. 83–99) shows that neighbouring varies according to the length that a community has been established, how physically close to each other's houses potential neighbours might be, age and stage of the life cycle (people with young families and elderly people being most involved) and gender (women's networks form around the house, men's around social life and work). He argues on the basis of his studies of informal neighbouring in the late 1970s and early 1980s that the political and social myth of mutual caring by neighbours comes from a time when housing was much more closely cramped together and their were few alternative services to provide help. So, he says, changes in society which have created greater social distance and privacy make the re-creation of such a pattern of care an impossible dream. Moreover, the absence of services and social distress implied by a return to this pattern of life make it positively undesirable. Abrams *et al.* (1989, p. 10) suggest that in acknowledging the importance of informal care as the main provider of social care. Conservative government ministers propose a role for the statutory services as a minimal, last-resort safety net.

Workers might seek to stimulate contacts with neighbours for the same reasons that contacts with friends might be encouraged: it provides a kind of social contact (although not with the intimacy of friendship) and some practical help might result. Except in a crisis, personal help of a more intimate kind is unlikely. Abrams (Bulmer, 1986, pp. 105 *et seq.*) explains this pattern of response by seeing neighbouring relationships as characterised by reciprocity. Neighbours help out in return for equal 'gifts' in return. However, Abrams argues that 'altruism' is a special kind of reciprocity, because all neighbouring carers gained an inexpressible benefit from being helpful to their neighbours.

Can informal care be made available?

Some answers to this question will already be apparent from the previous discussion. The kind of care available from neighbours and friends is likely to be relatively social, and relatively impersonal.

Personal care or 'tending' is likely to be available only from relatives, and generally only from female relatives or spouses.

If this is so, we must ask whether such female care is likely to be available. There are two reasons for doubting its availability. One is that the size of families is reducing, and the other is that more women are going out to work and are less available to care.

> Applying demographic trends to an 'average' family, David Eversley has estimated . . . that a hypothetical married couple age 85 and 80 in 1980, married in 1920, would, in 1980, have had forty-two female relatives alive, fourteen of whom would not have been working. By comparison, a married couple age 55 in 1980, married in 1950, would, by the year 2005, when they will have reached the age of 80, have only eleven female relatives alive, only three of whom would not be working. (Bulmer, 1987, p. 2)

The other major issue in making informal care available is the personal costs laid upon the carers. These can be extensive, but one study in Wales showed that carers felt most strongly about lack of privacy and loss of freedom. For women, conflict between different caring roles was a problem (Jones, 1993). Various studies identify restrictions in normal social life, high levels of suress, physical costs such as sleepless nights, illness, and economic losses because carers give up jobs, or do not accept promotion or changes in their jobs if they interfere with the caring task. Many of these aspects of caring are summarised in the term *burden* – either *caregiving burden* (Braithwaite, 1990) or *family burden* (Perring *et al.*, 1990). Braithwaite (p. 19) identifies three aspects of burden in long-term caring:

- *workload* – including the demands of the caring task (such as lifting, supervising, decision-making), and social–emotional demands (such as maintaining social networks and personal and emotional support);
- *resources* – including the coping strategies used, personality (such as self-esteem), health, availability of social support, financial well-being; and
- *crises of decline* – including the awareness that decline is continuing and death may be approaching, unpredictability, time constraints, the relationship between carer and receiver and the amount of choice in their lives which is restricted by the caring arrangement.

Braithwaite (1990, pp. 147–8) argues that many sources of burden are subjective. The feeling of burden is affected by how prepared, how responsible, how pressurised the carer is. Even where there is a family, many carers are mainly doing the job on their own as primary carers, even if there is a certain amount of help from others. A psychological study (Orbell *et al.*, 1993) found that two negative features about caring – care work strain and dissatisfaction with the relationship with the person being cared for – were in tension with two positive aspects – care work satisfaction and care lifestyle satisfaction. Stress was more likely to be experienced if the negative factors were strongly evident in any particular situation. This study suggests focusing on reducing these two negative aspects, so that the positives can be experienced more easily by carers. An important early American study (Collins and Pancoast, 1976) showed the importance of people in the community who local people naturally turn to, and argues that identifying them and supporting them in their efforts is more effective than trying to create forms of care which may be unacceptable.

Another important aspect of making caring available is the financial costs of caring. Glendinning (1992) found in a small survey of carers that most carers living alone with the cared-for person had very low incomes, because of the costs of caring, because they had given up jobs, or could only work part-time, and because social security benefits were linked to the cared-for person's benefit and householder status, which often did not take account adequately of the needs of the carer. In the long-term, because savings were being eaten up, older carers were likely to have lost so much that they would be in poverty in their own old age. Bytheway's (1989) study of older people in Wales shows how difficulties with health and practical problems are felt more powerfully because they are compounded by a constant struggle to maintain a supply of basic financial resources. Gillian Parker (1992) found that caring burdens were increased by spouses who were carers because they could not share the burden with others; the wish for privacy prevented their involving friends and neighbours. Her (1993) studies have shown how important marriage is in coping with disability. However, the extent to which couples were able to negotiate some degree of independence for the disabled partner reflected power relationships in the marriage before disability affected it, and existing attitudes to the opposite sex. Often disabled women were further disadvantaged by being denied any value in a situation where they were unable to play traditional female roles, and these were taken away from them. Often, needs were concealed from outsiders in order to maintain an impression that the disabled partner was not so dependent as was actually the case. Workers becoming involved in situations where disabled people are being cared for by their partners need to be aware of possibly complex interactions between conventional assumptions about social roles and the changes effected by increasing dependence.

From this account, it is evident that the availability of informal care is likely to become increasingly limited, and policies based on its availability are likely to be futile. Brenton (1985) argues that the Kent Community Care Scheme explicitly relies on the availability of female unemployed people, and Abrams *et al.*'s (1989) study of neighbourhood caring schemes shows that the availability of volunteer neighbourhood carers varied largely with the employment problems of the area and the availability of surplus workers.

The issue of the burden of caring draws attention to the neglect of support for carers. Richardson *et al.* (1989) set out a statement of need which applies to many carers and is endorsed by representative organisations:

- carers' own needs and contribution should be explicitly recognised;
- services should be tailored to individual circumstances, theirs as well as those of the cared-for person;
- services should be organised to reflect awareness of different cultural, racial and religious values;
- opportunities for long and short breaks from caring;
- practical help;
- someone to talk to, who meets their own emotional needs;
- information about services and benefits which could help;
- an income which covers the costs of caring and does not force carers into taking a job or sharing care when they do not want to;
- the chance to explore alternatives to family care; and
- consultation about services provided.

If these are carers' needs, then, what services can be made available to provide for them?

Support for informal care

The official guidance on carers' services (Haffenden, 1991) emphasises three basic aspects of provision:

- identifying and providing the right type of service for carers, by working with carers to find out precisely what they want, getting regular feedback from them about how the service is meeting their needs and being prepared to change things in accordance with the feedback;
- promoting the service, so that carers know about it, understand what it is trying to provide and that it is of good quality and can see how it might meet their needs; and
- making it a personal service, with the minimum of rules and regulations, good flexibility and a friendly and welcoming aspect.

The official guidance (Haffenden, 1991) then discusses examples of services according to the 'statement of need' identified above. Some examples involve 'self-help' by a group of people who share a problem. A parents' group organised a baby-sitting service for children with learning difficulties, flexibly, so that it met their precise needs. One area set up a family support centre for Asian families with physically disabled children. Attendants to provide respite for carers of elderly people with a physical or mental disability, and short-term respite care at volunteers' houses are other examples. Many areas set up carers' centres, so that carers could share experiences and gain some social life, information and access to services from an identifiable place. Hills (1991), evaluating the DoH demonstration projects, notes that these were well-received, as was counselling where it was directly related to the needs of the people being cared for. However, carer-run services and volunteer services often fell foul of the existing stress on carers and volunteers were only useful for less-intensive caring tasks. Schemes where host families provided respite care proved difficult because hosts were hard to find, and sometimes carers resented their being paid when carers received little financial help. Services where ordinary people were paid to provide care to relatives or neighbours revealed that there was a tension between the wish to overcome the inflexibilities of formally organised care, by stimulating informal resources to fill the gaps, but as soon as this becomes managed and controlled, it becomes less attractive to those involved, and the small-scale payment may be an insufficient compensation (Leat and Gay, 1987). This is what makes it so difficult to convert (as discussed above) informal networks into organised support.

Twigg *et al.* (1990) identify five types of service which may be offered:

- services aimed at the carer, mainly to relieve the pressures of caregiving and help manage emotional stress
- help for practical tasks
- providing relief from caring
- helping the carer to get more from the care system
- improving the level and quality of services to the cared-for person.

This typology helps workers to identify a number of focuses so that services that they plan might help support informal care, and thus maintain clients at the low end of the community care tariff. It also helps provide a useful assessment guide to see what needs might be met.

We must now turn to the skills necessary to work with informal carers in the client's network to fit those services to the needs identified.

Skills in care planning – negotiating in clients' networks

Negotiation has always been regarded as an important skill in social work, but it is a neglected one. One reason for the neglect may be that it is difficult to train people, because it involves several different roles, which are hard to simulate, so in training workers are plunged into the deep end during placements. Another reason may be that negotiation is associated with business, or international peacemaking, rather than the social services, and the literature is hard to convert.

The most important reason for the neglect of negotiation, however, is probably that as a concept it goes against the fundamental basis of traditional therapeutic social work. Negotiation assumes that a worker is in an equal position with the person that they are negotiating with, or at least that they have an equal right to contribute to the resolution of the issue that they are dealing with. Therapeutic social work tends to assume that workers are experts or have an official position which puts them in a position of 'advising' or 'helping'. The skills of interaction between human beings are similar, however.

Negotiation and community care

The 'equal-position' aspect of negotiation makes it an important skill in care planning, because the aim is to get several people within the client's network to contribute resources to their care. This means that they must be treated with respect as collaborating colleagues, rather than, as is often regrettably the case, disrespectfully as clients. Moreover, although we must not deny the social worker's professional and personal power, community care policy does not accord the care planner power to command resources from any source, and certainly not from informal carers. Is negotiation, then, the appropriate skill for gaining resources from within clients' networks to contribute to their care?

At first, it appears not so, because understanding of negotiation comes from a conflictual tradition. In this view, negotiation is a process by which people or groups pursue their interests, and the outcome divides the advantages between them, according to the circumstances that they are in conflict about, their relative power, and the skill with which they carry on the negotiation. This is called, 'distributive bargaining' – that is, it distributes the outcome among the parties.

There are some objections to formulating negotiation like this, which lead to an understanding of how it can be relevant to complex negotiations by care planners creating packages of care. First, this view of negotiation presumes that people are in conflict and will always pursue their own interests. In fact, they have a shared interest in completing the negotiation and coming to a resolution. They therefore have an interest in the opposing party's interests as well as their own. Pursuing a co-operative strategy in which all parties win, rather than all or some losing, is more appropriate. Feminist critics of the 'win–lose' approach to negotiation, often regard it as male 'game-playing'. Some writers (for example, Leritz, 1991) argue that it is better to negotiate so that both sides gain advantages (a 'win–win' situation – Morgan, 1987). Gray (1989) argues that we should seek to collaborate in the 'constructive management' of disagreements.

Pruitt and Rubin (1986) propose that negotiation can usefully be seen according to a *'dual-concern'* model as an interaction between concern for our own outcomes and concern for those of the other party. High concern for our own *and* the other's outcomes will lead us to problem-solving. Concern about our own, but not the other's, outcomes would lead to contending. Relationships between the parties, especially if these will continue after the negotiation, and a feeling of accountability to each other will also tend to lead to co-operative, problem-solving behaviour, rather than contending. These ideas are useful for social workers, since usually they will have a concern for the interests of other people whom they are trying to help, rather than or as well as their own. One situation in which this may not be true is where resource or managerial pressures divorce them unreasonably from concern for their clients' interests. They are also likely to have continuing relationships with clients and their carers and a feeling of accountability towards them or for them. All these lead to the suggestion that a problem-solving rather than contending approach to negotiation is most appropriate.

Another objection to the 'distributive bargaining' view of negotiation is that negotiators are not always sure of their interests, or of where they want to end up. For people in these positions, negotiations are much more of an 'exploration' of an unknown territory or a shared attempt to solve a problem than a 'game' between two partners. A further objection is that much of the skill in negotiation lies in effective communication rather than in the content of the interests or conflict resolution (Putnam and Roloff, 1992). This leads to a view that 'integrative bargaining' in which the parties co-operate to find a shared and accepted resolution of their problems is most appropriate for complex situations such as those that social workers are involved in.

Social context affects how negotiations take place. Social norms, for example, sometimes prevent conflict altogether by setting up social conventions, they regulate the way conflicts are carried on (for example, by inhibiting violence) and can resolve a dispute by providing a conventional solution.

Negotiating with informal carers

Building on this brief account of negotiation in theory, some approaches to negotiation with informal carers, actual or potential, within clients' networks can be identified. Care planners are likely to want to use a shared 'problem-solving' rather than contending approach. This will mean engaging carers in a joint decision-making process, encouraging a feeling of trust, making power relationships clear (that is, saying what can and cannot be done by the agency and the network) since clarity in power relationships adds to co-operative behaviour, and encouraging positive working relationships.

As with all social work activities, negotiation benefits from careful *preparation*. Workers need to explore the possible options and their pros and cons, and to find out about possible participants in the care plan and their possible roles, and things which may obstruct them in playing a part and things which may help them. An idea of the timescale is also important: is urgent resolution needed, is there an immovable obstacle which produces a time limit, or is there plenty of time to explore and perhaps try out different approaches to the problem? Another useful preparation may be to undertake some activities with the participants, or some of them, at the start. This is because trust and positive relationships build on past success, so that if the worker can start off by resolving one or two minor problems or providing some useful services at the outset, others are more likely to trust the genuineness of their efforts in the negotiation. An example is when the lone carer of an elderly lady in their own home seeks residential care, but this seems an excessive response. While engaging in discussions with the carer and others, the worker might provide some home help service, or an occasional night sitter, to allow the carer some respite while the investigation of possibilities goes on.

Establishing a problem-solving relationship involves creating an understanding among the people involved that they are dependent on each other for a resolution. The worker needs to make clear that he or she cannot do everything for the client, but will try to make a contribution, and that the purpose of working together is to bring together several contributions and try to make them work together. All the participants in the caring network are *interdependent*.

Another aspect of setting up the caring network is to identify and establish suitable means of communication. This may involve regular meetings, or arrangements to telephone each other, see each other as they pass on responsibilities (for example, a handover meeting) or leave written messages. Joint records, perhaps kept by the client, may be another important part of communication.

The style of communication may be important, too. Useful guidelines from the negotiation literature are summarised by Pruitt and Carnevale (1993):

- concentrate on the problem rather than the people involved;
- when people are being emotional, other people should try to be rational;
- when people are misunderstanding and getting confused, others should try to be sympathetic and understanding;
- consult everyone affected, even though they are not concentrating at present (because they will resent not being consulted afterwards);
- when people are being manipulative or deceptive, this can be openly acknowledged, but others should be honest and open rather than trying to pay them back in their own coin;
- where others are trying to apply pressure, try to avoid coercing them;
- especially when trying to persuade others, people should demonstrate being open to persuasion;
- when others are rejecting your contribution, try to be caring and open to learning from them;
- keep communication channels open;
- listen actively and respond to what is heard;
- be open about concern for others;
- be willing to change your ideas and open to change which benefits solving the problem;
- look again at your own interests that others cannot accept to see if they really are essential to you; if not, be prepared to change;
- reward people who make positive moves;
- do favours, encourage social easing, by sharing refreshments and taking part in social niceties; and
- locate and develop bonds between the people involved, however remote these might be.

In essence, all these ideas model to the others a positive attitude to the problem and to problem-solving.

Within such a relationship, it is useful then to explore all aspects of the problem that people involved can identify, hiding nothing even though it seems to get in the way, because it will still get in the way even when hidden, and hiding it will seem untrustworthy or as if you are not recognising a problem that someone has raised. This will tend to exclude them. It is useful to identify problems that are resolved or which can be easily dealt with, since this emphasises that the issues being faced are not insoluble, and are not overwhelming, but contain many positive aspects.

In looking for resolutions of problems, it is useful in principle to keep all the options open until all the problems are resolved. By starting with some issues and resolving them, people involved can have a sense of making progress, but this should be regarded as an interim resolution until everything is resolved. This comes from two essential principles of negotiating, to *keep options open*, and *maintain manoeuvrability*. Part of resolving the problems in a care plan requires identifying people's roles and tasks within the plan. Definitions of these should be specific. It may also be necessary to consider the time structure of the implementation of the roles and tasks.

Once all issues are resolved, the plan can be formally created. It may seem overpowering in many cases to create a written agreement, but this can be couched in the form of a timetable. Sometimes the advantage of a written agreement is that it emphasises the advantages gained for various people, in return for their contributions. One advantage to be clearly identified is where people are free of a responsibility or demand, as a result of the plan. The plan will also require arrangements for monitoring. This can also be encouraging for participants because it means that there is a clear point at which they can review, and possibly change, their commitment. They are thus not committing themselves for all time, and they know that their needs will be explicitly considered again at an agreed time. This can be an important reassurance to someone who is doubtful about taking something on.

Endword: planning and implementing the plan

In this chapter, we have been exploring the creation of a care plan. Central to the approach described here is seeing care planning as a process whereby the worker develops and uses personal relationships with clients, carers and other people who might become involved to strengthen commitment to and participation in the plan. This social work approach, using traditional social work skills, establishes the continuing relationship as the 'glue' which holds the plan and its elements together. The aspects of enabling, supporting and protection, whether seen as part of the process of identifying and formulating the plan or as a social work service offered as part of the plan itself, form an essential part of using social work throughout care management.

Post-Griffiths community care policy establishes an implicit tariff in which informal care is the preferred starting point. Exploring informal care, we found many conceptual and practical problems to bringing it into an organised package of services because of its essentially personal nature. However, we have seen that most care is provided informally, and it is crucial not to ignore it, since informal carers have many important needs which require support; if they are supported, the tariff presumes that informal care will be strengthened.

The initial part of creating a care package will involve negotiating within the client's existing network of informal carers and social contacts, and we finally explored ways of negotiation which are appropriate to community care in the social and health services. It is at this point that the 'client' reaches the point of becoming a service 'user', since to their assessed personal needs, to the social work basis of their care plan and to the informal network of care which they already received and which may be supported, we must now attach the formal services which will substitute for or provide that support. These services are the focus of the next chapter.

6

Implementing Care Plans

This chapter is concerned with *formal care*, that is, services organised separately from the personal networks of people needing care, fitting these services with informal care and making the whole package work together. The community care tariff emphasises the importance in post-Griffiths community care policy of starting from a basis in informal care. However, people seeking assessment hope also to receive services to add to their resources. Social work skills are the link and the 'glue' which hold packages of informal and formal services together. Bayley (1973) calls this 'interweaving'. It creates the 'seamless' service of community care policy from an accumulation of differently-administered services.

The social work role in this relates to the 'social care planning' or community social work aspect of social work, identified in Figure 1.1 (p. 2). Looking at this again in Figure 6.1, we can see how this inter-relates with other social work and care management roles. The community social work role focuses on developing new caring organisations and promoting their involvement and that of other community resources in effective caring activities. This is a developmental role, involving community organisations, and linking them with developmental resources from agencies. Community care policies, however, base this role on the needs and wishes of users and carers, and the community social work role overlaps with the counselling/ therapeutic role in promoting that involvement. Similarly, post-Griffiths community care policy requires caring organisations to be linked to the care planning and contracting processes in the care management system. Within care management, users and carers need to be helped to link effectively with care organisations.

Implementing a care plan starts, then, from developing the client's

Figure 6.1 *The three community care roles of social work, showing elements of the community social work role*

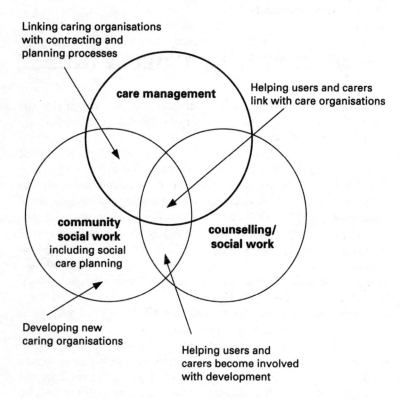

informal resources with formal services. There are two aspects to this, both involving carers and users in the process:

● linking and contracting with existing formal services
● creating new resources from community facilities.

The skills involved include linking and collaborative work between agencies and professionals, and community and development work in the community. These two areas of skill are the main focus of the last two sections of this chapter. The next section, however, is concerned with the range of services which are potentially available in community care services.

Community care services

Post-Griffiths community care policy assumes that services will be offered by a range of providers. One (not particularly helpful) way of understanding services is to identify various 'sectors' of provision: we met the 'informal' sector in Chapter 5. The formal sectors are:

- *public* services, provided by social services departments, health authorities (district health authorities, health service trusts, and contractors to family health services authorities such as general practitioners) and other departments of the local authority (housing and education being perhaps the most important);
- *voluntary sector* services, offered by charities, not-for-profit agencies and by community organisations;
- *private* services, offered by individuals or private companies, similar to the voluntary sector, but distributing their profits to their owners.

The last two sectors together are sometimes called the 'independent' sector.

At one time, these sectors could have been regarded as fairly distinct, and the role of the independent sector as fairly minimal, with the private sector virtually absent. The succession of events discussed in Chapter 2, however, the 'contract culture' of the mixed economy of care and the government's 'management approach' of creating a mixed economy of care, has made the differences indistinct. Virtually any service *may* be provided for a local authority by independent organisations on contract, and volunteers and carers can receive some funding to support their work. In some places services which were managed by the local authority have been hived off to independent companies. The local authority regulates the quality of the independent sector through registration and inspection, and by the quality control mechanisms in its contracts. The planning system for community care also involves representatives of all sectors (and users and carers).

Twigg *et al.* (1990) identify services which support carers in carrying out their caring responsibilities, and their account provides a useful summary of provision relevant to the first priority in the community care tariff.

- *Support groups (including centres) and information services* These include self-help groups of users and carers; similar groups associated with a general-purpose community centre or other services, such as a day centre or hospital; training and educational provision for users or carers; therapy groups and groups developed and perhaps run by professionals.
- *Help with domestic tasks and personal care* This includes domestic help agencies, the local authority home help service or volunteers. Voluntary schemes also provide routine services such as befriending, visiting and shopping, often with some emotional support. Respite schemes and night sitting or other 'care attendant' schemes also exist. More sophisticated and intensive, but still basically practical, 'homemaking' services are valued by clients, and helpful in reducing problems experienced by clients in the community (for example, see Cheetham, 1993). 'Meals on wheels' services and luncheon clubs offer meals to people unable to cook for themselves and some social contact. Community nursing services from the health authority or health care trust may offer bathing and other physical forms of care, such as surgical or other dressings. General practitioners and associated services provide medical care. 'Incontinence' services for people who cannot control urination or defecation fully include laundry, provision of incontinence protection and some emotional support and practical advice.
- *Respite care* This relieves limitations on carers' ordinary life and provides stimulation and change for the people being cared for. This may include day care (occupation and social interaction with others of a similar age or client group, together with some personal and medical care). Day care may also have social or medical therapeutic and treatment objectives, and training and education objectives, especially but not only for users with learning difficulties. Sometimes respite care is also provided in institutions, such as residential care homes or hospitals: usually this offers brief stays for 'holiday' purposes, but occasionally there are schemes for people to spend a high proportion, such as a half or a third of their time, in this form of care. It enables them to build up strength or receive regular treatment while still feeling that their base is at home. Many areas also have family placement schemes for people with disabilities or learning difficulties, or elderly people, where people with care needs are

placed permanently or temporarily with families offering care and involvement in their home life so substituting for an isolated or pressurised existence.

In addition to services in support of informal carers, there are a number of services provided directly to people with needs.

- *Social work or medical treatment*   This could be for physical or emotional difficulties.
- *Practical guidance and support in daily living and in dealing with other agencies, or in personal relationships, and for dealing with particular difficulties*   Examples are interpretation for people who are deaf or deaf-blind or training in mobility or in Braille or Moon for people who are blind or partially sighted. This may be particularly necessary for people with learning difficulties or who are recovering from physical traumas or mental illnesses being discharged from long-stay institutions.
- *Aids to mobility or other aspects of life and adaptations to premises which will enable people with disabilities to manage their lives as they would wish*   Among the possibilities are 'staying put' projects which help older people adapt and repair their homes, thus reducing the effect of housing pressures on the need to move into care (Leather and Mackintosh, 1993).
- *Education and opportunities for social experience*   These may not have been available either because of the help users need, or because of exclusion from limited ordinary provision or because they have special needs to be met. Examples include group holidays; financial and practical help for independent holidays; opportunities to take part in normal adult, further and higher education or special provision; social clubs or involvement in ordinary social provision or financial support for it.
- *Housing or living accommodation, and adaptations to living accommodation or other provision which allow people with care needs to live more independent lives*   Housing is sometimes linked with nearby housing, and day care or staff support made available in the locality, forming a dispersed housing scheme.
- *Transport to enable elderly or disabled people meet others and take part in life more actively*
- *Social security and other financial assistance and help with claiming rights or taking up opportunities*   The disabled living

allowance and other attendance allowances have complex claiming
conditions and the government is trying to restrict the cost of
the scheme. However, they are useful ways of increasing income to give users flexibility in buying services.

● *Participation in political and social structures and opportunities
  to influence decisions that effect the service user.*

It is impossible to review the huge range of literature which relates
these services to specific client groups. Useful summaries are contained in:

● Twigg *et al.* (1990) – on services for carers;
● Lynch and Perry (1992), Smith *et al.* (1993) and Robbins (1993)
  – on the whole range of community care clients;
● Patmore (1987), Pilling (1991), Sherlock (1991), Weller and
  Muijen (1993) – on services for people with long-term mental
  illness;
● Sinclair *et al.* (1990) and Day (1993) – on older people;
● Towell (1988), Brigden and Todd (1993) – on people with learning
  difficulties; and
● Harrison, J. (1987) – on people with physical disabilities.

There are, moreover, publications which provide a practical account
of setting up particular services, such as Carol Robinson (1991) on
respite care for disabled or older people. Studies of the problems of
particular groups of clients with long-term care needs also provide
indications of the kinds of services that could usefully be provided.

Ferlie *et al.* (1989), as part of a survey of a variety of local services for elderly people, argue that without providing services themselves, public agencies could take a more active role in promoting
co-ordinating work in a variety of agencies; use public funding to
provide incentives for voluntary organisations to co-ordinate their
efforts with each other and public sector services; and train and
develop support for private sector organisations so that they relate
more effectively to the whole range of services. They argue that a
more active role for SSDs in seeking efficiency within the system,
rather than being reactive to outside agencies' demands, would bring
dividends.

Sinclair *et al.* (1988) surveyed elderly people living alone. They
suggest that simple provision could improve the quality of life for

people living alone. Examples are a service which could stand in for neighbours when they went away; plans for making links with people who visited older people living alone (most people living alone received such visits); modern alarm and communication systems in case there was an accident; and transport to see friends and encouragement to neighbours, perhaps through payments from attendance allowances.

The demands of aware service users and the assumptions of post-Griffiths community care policy suggest a need to consider care needs and clients in particular ways; in particular an empowering, social model of the problems which are being dealt with. Characteristics of the approach include the following.

● *Normalisation or social role valorisation* This approach originated in work with people with learning difficulties in Scandinavia (Emerson, 1992). Its aim was to enable people with learning difficulties to experience patterns of life as close as possible to those of 'ordinary' people. The focuses of such patterns of life include the rhythm of the day, week and year, so that normal meal, work, leisure and holiday times are acknowledged; an ordinary life cycle, including changes in lifestyle associated with adulthood and possibly marriage; self-determination and involvement in decision-making about lifestyle; ordinary provision for claiming social security benefits and receiving wages; and a living environment which is similar to ordinary housing. A Canadian, Wolfensberger (1972), and the British Campaign for People with Mental Handicaps, developed and applied the ideas. Wolfensberger (1984) developed the concept of 'social role valorisation' to refer to the need to arrange services to provide people with learning difficulties with the opportunity to take up roles in society which would be generally socially valued. Related to normalisation there are tools for evaluating services for people with learning difficulties: PASS (Program Analysis of Service Systems) and PASSING (Program Analysis of Service Systems Implementing of Normalisation Goals).

● *Normal life models of service provision* (Towell, 1988) These have developed from normalisation ideas in the UK, extending into employment and housing provision. Williams and Tyne (1988) suggest that among the devaluing experiences to be avoided are physical segregation and isolation from socially valued people;

lack of roots and relationships; insecurity and lack of control over living arrangements; lack of chances to gain new experiences; awareness of being a burden to others; and feeling that life is wasted. To redress these common experiences among users of services, they suggest services should offer facilities that give easy access to a variety of people and places not close to many others who seem 'odd', with comfortable settings in which service users are treated well as individuals. In the housing field, the view emphasised (Bayliss, 1987) seeing people as residents rather than patients or clients, having rights to security of tenure, involvement in management, choice in how they managed their daily lives, choice over fellow residents and privacy in shared housing. Even 'challenging behaviour', such as violence or aggression, should not lead to rejection but to forming services which help people to manage their behaviour appropriately (Maher and Russell, 1988).

- *Empowerment as a philosophy in management and social care* In social care the philosophy contains several elements, according to Adams (1990). It implies self-management by service users; handing over power, for example by being open about information; being against bureaucratic forms of organisation and avoiding unnecessary organisational requirements of service users; emphasising co-operation between users, carers and professionals; and emphasising the shared experience of users. In a more political analysis, Solomon (1976) emphasises the importance of helping people overcome barriers which are established by past experience of powerlessness in their capacity to deal with problems in their lives. Rees (1991) similarly identifies the 'biography' of the experiences of powerlessness as an essential element to explore within social work and emphasises the complex interactions of different aspects of power, which can be both helpful and hindering. Also crucial in his view is the use of language as an expression of power and oppression.

- *Anti-discriminatory practice* Similar ideas underlie the importance of anti-discriminatory practice (Thompson, N., 1993). Identifiably different groups in society experience discrimination because of their difference which means that inequalities in power oppress them and exclude them from full involvement in society. Workers need to understand and recognise features of the services which they represent that participate in these social processes, seek to reduce their effect on service users and avoid behaving in ways which reinforce or extend such oppressions. It is an assumption of these ideas that such forces are always present in social structures and cannot be fully eliminated, although they can be combated and their effects mitigated.

- *Social rather than medical models of disability have become more important* (Oliver, 1990) A medical model of disability concentrates on the impairment in a disabled person's physical condition, as compared with a 'normal' person. This then leads them to be unable to perform ordinary actions, and requires treatment to improve their functioning, or if possible restore normality. The social model identifies the fact that the disability derives from social definitions of what is normal, and this leads the world to be organised in ways which fit the conventional pattern of functioning. So, the reason why someone confined to a wheelchair finds it difficult to get around is that roads and buildings are not designed to provide for wheelchair users; if they were, the consequences of the disability would be less great. Related to this are social attitudes. People regard the 'normal' condition as desirable, and this tends to reject valued aspects of the disabled person's experience, to treat their disability as a 'personal tragedy' or to blame them for their inadquacies. For example, profoundly Deaf people who have been so from birth regard themselves as part of a community with its own culture and language (thus it is given a capital 'D'; people outside the community are merely deaf). Thus, pity for being Deaf is inappropriate, since in many ways this is a valued state; by extension efforts to 'cure' deafness by medical technology can be regarded as an attack on cultural values of the Deaf community.
- *The independent living movement (Morris, 1993b) not only proposes that disabled people should live independently but that they should be provided with facilities to do so* It also says that, because all human life is valuable, rather than having services controlled by others, disabled people should be given the money to enable them to buy services which they can control themselves, making their own choices and participating fully in society (Morris, 1993b, p. 21). Thus, rather than being given a home help, they should receive the equivalent in money, and be enabled to employ their own help. Since many people do not want to be bothered by the bureaucracies of becoming employers,

services run by disabled people or voluntary organisations on
the principle of control by the person in need may be an appropriate half-way house. Brown and Ringma (1989) describe a small-
scale shared residential home or organised on the basis of the
resident as employer; issues such as where friendships and sexual
relationships might arise between resident and worker need, in
their view, constant negotiation.

● *The political economy model of ageing emphasises how our view
of people in later life is 'socially constructed' by views of ageing* (Laczko and Phillipson, 1991)   Because older people do not
make a contribution in the labour market and may become more
dependent, particularly on state services, they may be seen as
having little social value. Moreover, our high valuation of youth
may lead us to deny sexual and social needs, and ignore or
ghettoise leisure and social facilities for older people who cannot afford high-cost private leisure facilities aimed at young people.

Some of these approaches conflict with each other, in some re-
spects. For example, 'normalisation' implies a high valuation of conventional views on 'normal' which some perspectives discussed here
would reject (Szivos, 1992). There are also different conceptions of
normalisation. Szivos (1992) argues that some views accept and regard
difference positively (enabling more group and mutual support) than
Wolfensberger's view, which tends to be oriented towards treating
and 'improving' people's functioning. It may be better to help people
develop a positive social identity including their disability, as independent living models seek to do. Critics note that some of these
approaches contain 'radical romantic' ideals of socially stigmatised
groups as always the victims of society's evils. Such views can
also lead to the rejection of efforts to improve individual problems
(for example, treatment for deafness), because it is 'society's' fault
that these are seen as problems. However, the fact that, say, a man
with severe cerebral palsy can live an independent life, communicate with others, marry, work and have a socially satisfying life
does not negate the gains that preventing the condition might bring,
and searching for treatment should not devalue the life led by someone
with a disability.

It is important, therefore, to avoid slipping into seeing people as
always passive victims, while taking advantage of the social perspectives on definitions and reactions to the needs which commu-

nity care services deal with, so that people are seen as self-acting, and so that we value their existing lifestyle and achievements rather than comparing these inappropriately with 'normality'. Community care policy, with its emphasis on cost-efficient service provision, might lead us to take the cheap option of institutionalising someone because we do not value what they get out of their independent lifestyle. Social perspectives on human needs nearly always usefully alert us to the barriers to good service that users experience and barriers to their own self-assertion that conventional views of them and their needs almost always imply.

One of the hopes of community care policy is that such barriers can be broken down by effective linking between services, and between the formal services and the informal network and users' needs which have been explored at the care planning stage of care management; and by developing new services in ways which are appropriate to needs of potential services users and respond to their wishes. These two aspects of implementing care plans are the focus of the next two sections.

Linking and collaborative work

Official guidance

Post-Griffiths community care policy is essentially about linking and collaboration between services. This is made clear in the Minister's introduction to the Policy Guidance:

> If implementation is to be effective, there must be close working links between all agencies – social services departments, NHS bodies, housing authorities and associations, voluntary organisations and private sector service providers. These working links must take full account of the views and needs of those being cared for and their carers.   (Bottomley, 1990)

The Policy Guidance emphasises the need for co-operation at the service development level of community care planning (para. 2.7) as required by Section 46 of the *NHS&CCA, 1990*. In particular there should be planning agreements between SSD's, district health authorities and family services authorities (which control independent contractors to the health service, such as general practitioners), which identify resources provided by each (para. 2.11–3). Regional health authorities and regional social services inspectorates are to help authorities to collaborate (para. 2.14). Authorities are supposed to be separately accountable for their performance, but their success in collaboration should be an aspect of evaluation of their success (para. 2.14). This guidance ignores the possibility of buck-passing, in which one blames their own failure on the failure of the other, which might not accept responsibility, or might reciprocate blame.

The next level of collaboration is at the care management level. Section 46(3) of the Act lays a legal duty on SSDs to assess for their own services, and Section 47(3) requires them to bring housing and health care needs to the attention of the relevant authorities. All should be involved in a joint assessment arrangement (DoH, 1990, paras 3.32–5). One person, usually the care manager, might assess on behalf of all of them, but for specialist assessments others might take on part of the assessment. Health authorities still have a legal duty to provide and assess for nursing care needs (paras 3.36–9).

The care management role in collaboration is set out in more detail in the Care Management and Assessment Guides (SSI/SWSG, 1991a and 1991b). One of the claimed 'ten key benefits' of care management is 'better integration of services within and between agencies' (SSI/SWSG 1991a, p. 13). Partnership with users and carers and greater continuity of care are also mentioned. The Managers' Guide (SSI/SWSG, 1991b, paras 4.9–12) sets out advice about inter-agency arrangements, and emphasises communication systems, standard referral and assessment systems and possibly joint databases. In addition, a good informal network of communication should reduce the need for large case conferences, and mutual trust and understanding and a common culture should be built up by joint training. The Practitioners' Guide (SSI/SWSG, 1991a, pp. 23–5) emphasises the importance of developing shared values and valuing the contributions of different agencies.

In the early stages, the Managers' Guidance (SSI/SWSG, 1991b, p. 24) assumes that it may be necessary to differentiate accountability for different aspects of the service clearly, but eventually joint provision and purchasing is hoped for. Drawing on PSSRU research, the guide (p. 24) advises developing clarity of roles and responsibilities, especially by joint documents; using joint mechanisms such as joint care planning teams to help develop and manage co-operation; and promoting individual contacts between managers to maintain allies and advocates in the other organisation. In particular, 'operational policies and clear accountability help to reduce conflict and confusion' (p. 79).

In this guidance, we see a tension between two aspects of collaboration: accountability through clear definition of distinct responsibilities and at the same time increasingly joint activity through shared values and policies. This partly seen as a matter of timescale (clarity firs, jointness later), but both aspects are assumed to be present throughout. Similarly, the responsibilities of agencies are clearly established, but co-operation and communication between individuals are to overcome difficulties. The discontinuities created by separation of agencies are to be overcome by individual co-operation and joint action. Is this a viable approach? It has never worked so far in health and social services co-operation.

Team, teamwork and collaboration

One significant approach to making the individual relationships work within the formally established structure of community care is *multidisciplinary teamwork*. This approach assumes that two different aspects of organisation can be brought together:

- *working in teams* – in which groups of staff working together develop or are helped to develop shared values and objectives, and shared working practices and priorities enabling the overall service that they provide to be better than it would be if they worked individually;
- *multi-disciplinary work* – in which groups of staff from different professional backgrounds, with different knowledge bases and values, are brought together to contribute their different areas of knowledge to the same service user or group of service users.

There are problems with both of these concepts, and putting them together extends the complexity of the issues. 'Teamwork' is an idealisation representing hope or expectation rather than an actuality (Payne, 1982). The *developmental* view of teamwork suggests that people working together will collaborate towards agreed ends, usually by a process of developing group relationships and shared values between them. The *contingency* view suggests, alternatively, that different forms of collaboration are appropriate to different situations, and the preferences of the participants, the demands of their work and the structure of the organisation within which they work. Øvretveit (1993) argues that we should not seek an ideal model of co-operation in groups of workers, but should develop 'workable' arrangements in localities, by recognising and overcoming barriers.

'Multi-disciplinary' work is one of a cluster of concepts, including 'multi-professional' and 'inter-disciplinary' which have slightly different meanings. It implies that several different kinds of people are working together, and their differences come from an academic and professional discipline; the idea of 'discipline' tends to emphasise theoretical or learning base, while 'professional' tends to emphasise the professional value system represented by different participants, though both ideas are clearly related. The idea of 'inter-disciplinary work' tends to emphasise working relationships and connections between the ideas and professions. 'Multi-professional work' seems to emphasise a more divided application of ideas in some co-operative venture. Multi-professional or inter-professional or disciplinary work should not be confused with multi-agency or inter-agency work. One agency might contain different occupational groups and therefore require internally multi-professional or inter-professional work. Multi-agency or inter-agency work might be between agencies containing the same occupational groups. These differences alert us to the fact that organisational, professional and disciplinary differences need to be evaluated and worked with.

One response to the difficulties of teamwork as a concept which might guide practice is to emphasise the variety of relationships which might be possible among people who work together. The coherent group with everyone working in one place seems only applicable to a small range of situations. This has led to emphasis on seeing relationships among different people working together as relatively loose or tight 'networks', and exploring the nature of them, rather than assuming that a group process is the most appropriate one. This helps in understanding multi-disciplinary work, since it is easier to conceive of networks operating across professional and organisational boundaries than to seek to develop group relationships across such boundaries (although this is sometimes possible and desirable). Networking among professionals is also a helpful concept in community care policy, because it links directly with understanding informal care as a process of working within the service user's personal network. The formal network involved in a case can then be conceived of as an aspect or extension of the user's informal network. The problem with this is that it emphasises the individualisation of work within community care, associated with the plans for each individual client of the services. In practice, this may be convenient, but it neglects the importance of the continuing professional networks. Because these are strongly established, the expectations of the people within them about how they will function is likely to be much more powerful than the needs of a particular client, if these are different from the conventions. This is another instance of where the individualisation within community care policy can prevent new patterns of service and practice from growing up.

Research on multi-disciplinary work has been strongly influenced by the work of Øvretveit (1993) in his consultancy-style work with a wide variety of health and social services teams, and two major projects on community mental handicap teams established in the 1980s in Wales (Grant *et al.*, 1986; McGrath, 1991) and England (Brown and Wistow, 1990).

Øvretveit (1993) shows that many problems of co-operation derive from organisational problems and 'perverse incentives' which inhibit co-operation, rather than from personality problems. He distinguishes between:

- *client teams*, the changing group of people brought together around a service user to provide the package of care;
- *network-association teams*, associations of service providers relating to each other to refer and co-ordinate work among themselves, and
- *formal teams*, working groups with defined membership, shared policies and a team leader.

Teams vary according to:

- *structure* – team membership and management, including connections to managers outside the team (Because there may be several different agencies represented in a multi-disciplinary team, there may be a number of management connections to be considered.)
- *integration* – the closeness of links between members; and
- *process* – how users are received, dealt with and passed among members of the team.

In looking at the management of teams, Øvretveit shows that team-work among the members becomes important at different stages. For example, in some single-agency teams the team decisions on who should work with the case are made after reception and intake. The members then work independently. Others use a teamwork process at several stages, for example in helping each other plan their work, or in reviewing cases. More generally, teams set priorities, and Øvretveit sets out a process by which this can usefully be done: the precise confines of the client groups involved in the priority-setting exercise; exploration of their needs to understand them better; exploration of the team's resources and views on those needs, including clarifying present use of resources; decisions about future responses and targets for making changes from the present practice to the future; and, finally, carrying out and then reviewing those decisions.

Another important aspect of teamwork is deciding on the tasks that team members undertake, which then form their roles within the team, and improving how those roles relate to one another. In essence, teamwork is a form of division of labour, a way of dividing up a task which is too big for one person (*task differentiation*), and then creating roles for the members which form sensible packages of responsibility (*role integration*) (Payne, 1982, pp. 50–6). Øvretveit (1993, pp. 113–120) suggests that there are several common problems in this process.

- *Poor or disputed co-ordination*   To deal with this, workers getting involved with a service user should check who the care manager or other key worker is, and if there is not one, should try to ensure that agreement is reached among the relevant agencies about who should act in this way.
- *De-skilling*   People can spend so much time on co-ordination and care management that they have no time for working with clients, and lose their skills in doing so. In effect, they get into a routine of organising services, without including the interpersonal aspects of working with users and carers in the way suggested as so important in Chapter 5. Also, working in a multi-disciplinary way can make workers feel that their essential disciplines are lost in the generality of the team's responsibility, or that it is contrary to good teamwork to develop and practise separate skills. Here it is important for teams to value difference as well as sameness. It is useful to identify explicitly through a joint

exercise and seek to use effectively both personal characteristics and general and professionally specific skills that individuals in the team have. Teamwork does not aim at sameness, but at the effective use of variety.

- *Contested role overlap* There may be arguments about duplication, gaps in provision (because two or several members *can* do the work, it does not mean that they *will* do so), or whether it is appropriate or wrong for one or other profession to carry out particular tasks. A useful approach here is to carry out an exercise for each occupational group to identity skills, knowledge and responsibilities specific to their profession, and those that are common (such as co-ordination skills and management skills and responsibilities, both as they see it and as they think others see it) and to share those perceptions. A debate about overlap can then develop.

- *Reduced role autonomy* Sometimes, people lose autonomy by being a team member in such a way that it prevents them from acting effectively. Psychologists, for example, are often pressed to do more therapeutic work, when they feel their skills are better suited to assessment or consultancy to others. Teams need to have explicit debates about issues of this kind, perhaps by sharing some case studies, and experimenting with different ways of working on similar cases to see how different approaches from those that they use now will work.

- *Role overload* Many teams face the problem of too much work of the wrong kind. Team members may also have to take on too many roles, which conflict or require too great a range of skills for them to undertake them effectively. Clear priority and referral schemes can help here, so that work can be stockpiled for referred on and team members supported in rejecting low-priority work.

An important aspect of role integration is helping team members to take on roles which are appropriate not to only their professional skills and experience but also to their personal knowledge, values and style. Belbin (1981) studied management teams in commercial settings and came up with a number of roles (such as 'monitor/ evaluator' or 'resource investigator') which team members seemed to play, which were unrelated to their work role and seemed to be a matter of personal style. He shows that the roles taken on are also to some extent variable, so that particular individuals may have a role in one situation and another elsewhere. People can also be developed in the performance of roles which are not pre-eminent in their existing style. Belbin also argues that roles interact or conflict with one another, and people should not be expected to pursue roles which are in opposition to or inconsistent with one another. On the other hand, teams which have a predominance of people who prefer a particular role or who have a role conspicuously absent may have difficulties in functioning well. One team I dealt with, for example, contained several completer-finishers (who are careful to check detail and ensure that tasks are properly completed before going on to the next), and lacked shapers and 'plants' (who help define objectives and are keen to explore new ideas). Everything was done to a high standard, but development of new projects and creativity was slow. There are tests or exercises which help teams explore these possibilities (Belbin, 1982; Platt *et al.*, 1988). Using these, it is possible to identify training options, or recruit new staff to fill gaps. Caution is needed in using Belbin's work, however, since he studied groups of people with management responsibilities, rather than those with direct service responsibilities, and because his work covers commercial rather than public service occupational groups. None the less, many people have found the ideas useful.

McGrath's research (1991) also identified the importance of management structures, clarity of professional role and, crucially, the importance of effective team leadership in enabling multi-professional work in a team to operate well. Arrangements between agencies involved also needed to support teamwork.

Organisational factors are particularly important when co-operating across sector boundaries, because people in the public sector, who are providing most of the care managers, may not have a good understanding of factors which affect voluntary and private sector organisations. In particular, my experience is that people with no experience in the independent sector have a poor understanding of the pressures of insecure finance, and the need to make sure that things are properly funded, and the consequences of relatively flexible but perhaps unsupportive or confusing management systems. Also, representative machinery and liaison between organisations in these sectors may not be strong. Value differences can also get in the way, for example, where public sector staff are hostile to the idea of making 'profits' from people in need, or private sector staff stereotype public sector organisations as bureaucratic and slow.

Lynch and Perry (1992, pp. 278–80), for example, exploring a number of independent community care projects run by voluntary organisations, found that clearly identified liaison workers in local authorities helped projects to build links and understanding. However, one difficulty was that project workers had local liaison workers to build links in working with service users and at the same time had liaison with senior staff in the commissioning side of health and social services authorities. This led to conflicts and unease in local relationships. Because funding and security depended on the commissioning agency, relationships around service provision could be tense, since where there were no block contracts, failure to use the service had consequences for survival.

Linking skills

Linking skills can be divided into four main groups:

- *liaison* – making and maintaining contact with other organisations or people;
- *co-ordination* – ensuring that organisations and people work in ways which support and complement each other's work;
- *representation* – acting on behalf of one agency or person in their relationships with another; and
- *presentation* – promoting and demonstrating understanding about your work with another person or organisation. (Payne, 1993a)

I have written more extensively about the practice of linking work elsewhere (Payne, 1993a). The important points are that it needs to:

- *be planned* – both in the case of an individual relationship and in the case of an agency or team considering its wider relationships;
- *consider interpersonal aspects of the link* – including power relationships and the fact that increases in involvement between people or organisations inevitably require an increase in intrusion into their decision-making; and
- *relate to the formal structures and financing of the agencies involved.*

Planning involves thinking about whether the link is needed at all; its aims; structuring it (how often contacts are made, what activities are involved, who will do what, the styles of behaviour that are appropriate); the use of resources; and controlling and reporting back about links, where these are on behalf of an organisation or group. For example, Mrs Falkner is an elderly lady who needs meals provided (by a social services meals on wheels service), some domestic help (by a private agency) and a check on her safety, with some element of social support (offered by a neighbour, who is to receive an honorarium). It would be unhelpful if the people providing these services all arrived at lunchtime; the contacts need to be spread through the day, and week, to offer maximum security and social contact. There is a risk that the neighbour, who is somewhat self-important, will see others' efforts at social support or reporting on Mrs Falkner's safety as intrusion into her area of work (thus perhaps placing the continuation of her honorarium at risk). On the other hand, the knowledge of the neighbour's involvement may make the domestic agency and the meals deliverers less alert to social needs or safety; meaning that fear of intrusion leads to lack of involvement (seeing involvement and intrusion as emotional states as well as actions). Careful planning of sequences of events, using a shared diary for example, and careful discussion of the extent and recognition of the value of overlap between roles will be important contributions by a social worker or care manager to making this package of care work well.

The objectives of linking work may be simply to avoid gaps and overlaps between organisations or individuals providing a service. However, it is possible to have greater ambitions, and Orme and Glastonbury (1993, pp. 45–50) argue that the implementation of community care policy requires changes that develop congruence between services and a shared set of values. In a particular case or more generally, it is possible to develop:

● *aligned strategies* – so that agreement is developed about objectives and common ways of organising work;
● *aligned attitudes and values* – so that people in different agencies or aspects of the service are likely to be mutually supportive and facilitative in their attitudes; and
● *integrated structures* between agencies or aspects of service, so that the organisational arrangements begin to support the interpersonal work.   (Payne, 1993a, p. 56)

An aspect of achieving these wider linking goals is the development of services or the service system which enhance the whole network of provision. This aspect of implementing care plans leads us into the community social work and social care planning role of social work within community care.

Community work, community social work and community care

One of the objectives of community care policy is to mobilise underused resources in the community: resources of the neighbourhood, of friends, colleagues and particularly relatives of people in need of care. Social work's classic methods for developing and involving community resources in helping derive from community work. In the 1970s and 1980s, ideas from community work were interpreted to form part of more conventional social work practice, through the evolution of community social work. To put ideas for mobilising community resources into context, therefore, we need to examine the relationship of community work and community social work to community care.

Community work has a long history as an aspect of social work, although it would not be regarded as only a form of social work, since training for it, the formation of its ideas and its practice have been somewhat separate from social work. The essential aspects of community work are that workers should help people with shared interests to come together, work out what their needs are among themselves and then jointly take action to resolve those needs. They might do this by working together to meet those needs, by developing projects which would enable the people concerned to gain support to meet them or by campaigning to ensure that they are met by those responsible – particularly public authorities in social matters, but also, in the case of consumer campaigns, by getting private companies to meet their responsibilities. The skills involved are partly in bringing together groups and enabling them to function well, but also in marketing, planning, management and campaigning at a broader level.

As stated, this looks innocuous. In practice, however, community work has proved controversial and problematic. Bringing people together tends to allow them to share concerns which relate to how they are dealt with by powerful organisations in their lives. It tends to be carried out in particularly deprived communities such as, for example, minority ethnic communities where power relationships oppress many in the community, and it draws attention to inequalities in service provision and in power which lie behind severe deprivation. Thus, much community work becomes a struggle between people in powerless positions against the powerful. This may feel defeating or exhilarating for those involved, but may not produce practice results for the problems they set out with. It may also lead governments to see this as trespassing from professional work into the political arena, and to be inappropriate for services provided by government. The identification of structural inequalities as the main issue in inner city areas, for example, led to the destruction of government community development projects in the 1970s. Where self-managed services do result, the pressures involved in management and financing can lead to demotivation and lack of further development.

None the less, local organisations and government can work together and local government can pursue *community development*. Broady and Hedley (1989) studied a number of attempts to do so in local authorities around Britain. They argue that while local authorities have an important role in providing services and taking a lead in planning, they are not the only bodies concerned with public welfare. In a pluralistic democracy, where electing a representative body does not give it exclusive rights to organise everything but should enable other groups to participate with it, authorities should set out to promote partnership. This should come from two directions, in Broady and Hedley's view. There should be attempts to enable groups to define issues that they identify and act to respond to them, in the traditional community work approach; and there should also be attempts to make local authority services more responsive to public needs. They identify a variety of ways in which such community development may be interpreted, which can be further expanded to reflect the needs of community care policy:

● *liaison with parish councils* – to promote responsiveness to local opinion; for community care this will involve a larger number of official and semi-official bodies, particularly in the health field;
● *providing facilities* – where neighbourhoods are isolated or bereft of community provision; for community care this might involve opening up meeting places in local buildings where user

and carer groups and other neighbourhood organisations can develop welfare provision;

- *decentralising facilities*; essential in community care if a truly local response to need is to be made;
- *self-management of buildings* – which enables local groups to be involved and to direct how facilities available to them are used; for community care this further encourages user and carer involvement, and may make facilities more responsive to their needs, by opening at unconventional hours. It may also mean a preparedness to use facilities in other people's ownership, which local authorities might not previously have used, such as pubs or shops;
- *consultation and participation in service-delivery* – integral to community care;
- *co-opting voluntary organisations to extend their own services* – also essential to community care policy;
- *local welfare planning* – on the assumption that involvement will lead to more effective facilities because people will be more prepared and able to use them;
- *general support for the voluntary sector* – by recognising its role in policy-making and provision by joint decision-making, thus strengthening the capacity of the sector to respond to demand and be creative in its own developments;
- *extending democracy by connecting decision-making to local representation by politicians* – in community care, the importance of facilitating participation on an equal basis by people who may be stigmatised or disadvantaged by the condition for which they are receiving care must include participation in democratic processes;
- *direct support of neighbourhood groups* – by supporting linking mechanisms for informal groups to get together and represent the needs of a neighbourhood.

This account of the variety of options shows that local authorities can offer valuable opportunities for community development within their areas in a positive and co-operative way with their citizens, while not denying the need for campaigning and conflict on occasions.

A similar attitude is evinced in *community social work*. This concept grew out of a number of efforts to make better contact with local needs and resources in SSDs after the local government re-

168 _Social Work and Community Care_

organisation of 1974 increased the size and remoteness of many local authorities. The basic ideas are set out in an early publication (Hadley and McGrath, 1980) as offering:

- teams based on local 'patches', smaller than conventional social services areas
- good information about the area
- accessibility and acceptability to local people
- good liaison with other local agencies
- integration of field and domiciliary workers
- participative management systems
- autonomy in local teams.

An important study (Hadley and McGrath, 1984) comparing two local teams in Wakefield showed that departments organised on this basis found out more about their area and were able to intervene more quickly, and with more flexible resources. Later studies elsewhere (for example, Bayley _et al._ (1987) showed similar results, in that departments were more knowledgeable about their area and its problems and liaised better with related agencies. However, outcomes in work with cases showed little appreciable change. This may be because so many other legal and administrative factors affect the general outcome of specific case activities in the social services.

   The Barclay Report (1982) on the role of tasks of social workers, espoused community social work, but there was concern that this might lead social work practice into the kind of generalised political conflicts which had surrounded community work in its more conventional form. There was also criticism that voluntary organisations (Payne, 1986b) and informal networks (Walton, 1986) would not be able to sustain the kinds of involvements that would be required to promote such work widely, and that this would divert them from wider purposes and community priorities towards meeting local authority and welfare priorities. Some departments began widescale moves towards implementing community social work in their areas. One, in East Sussex, was researched from different points of view (Hadley _et al._, 1984; Hadley and Young, (1990) Beresford and Croft, 1986). Although a more localised and responsive organisation resulted, there is doubt about whether users of the services noticed significant changes to the kind of services they received.

Genuine involvement in decision-making, either more generally or in particular cases, does not seem to have resulted. Developments have continued, particularly through the Practice and Development Exchange of the National Institute for Social Work (Smale *et al.*, 1988; Smale and Bennett, 1989; Darvill and Smale, 1990).

Some of the more grandiose statements about community social work (for example, Smale *et al.*, 1988) see it as a way of changing the organisational perspective of social services and the practice of social work. Barr (1989) contends that it is essential for the community ideology and responsiveness required by effective community social work to permeate the whole team, and the department, if the innovation is not to be marginalised or turned into the development of 'special' projects. Smale and Tuson (1990) argue that it can be a particularly relevant way of organising social services to provide community care services.

Some of the concerns of community care policy are foreshadowed in these issues around community social work. These include the wish to develop community responsiveness among social work teams and agencies; the involvement of carers and users in decisions which affect them and in planning and developing services; integration and liaison between services and authorities; and collaboration between workers through teamwork. Community social work also has concerns about the aspects of team management and workload in later formulations, which relate to Orme and Glastonbury's (1993) contention that workload management is crucial to care management.

The central conflict within community development is that between developing services and projects which respond to social services requirements, and promoting involvement in processes for community decision-making among people in particular areas or with shared interests, which may not reflect or may conflict with social services priorities. The evidence is that a degree of involvement in services and much better community responsiveness on the part of agencies can be developed. Genuine community influence or, to go further, control, may be much harder to achieve, even if it is desired. A distinction must also be drawn between the interests of the community as a whole and those of users and carers. There may be no interest in the particular needs of groups of users of community care services; priorities for other people may lie elsewhere. On the other hand, where links can be created with generalist community groups, there is the possibility that users can be more closely integrated into other community activities and participate in more general community decision-making and activity.

Henderson and Armstrong (1993) approach these issues by proposing that workers should use community work skills within community care services, while not regarding such activities as necessarily carrying out community work. Important aspects of a community work skills approach in community care are:

- *having concern for community interest* – and organising the team to think about broad community interests; regular review of local newspapers, attendance at local events;
- *knowing the physical area* – by travelling through it on foot and public transport, using local shops and getting to know local people;
- *gathering community information* – about resources and people in the community who have particular interests;
- *identifying shared interests and links between different clients and groups, and putting them in touch with one another* – this may involve being relatively open about the work being done on particular cases, so that others can see links;
- *offering resources to actual or potential local groups* – this may include the time of a worker, opportunities to use meeting space, a crèche for children so that parents can meet, sitting services so that carers can meet, office facilities such as photocopying, typing and mailing;
- *identifying and enabling the use of community facilities* – such as organisations, buildings and individuals and groups who can support one another;
- *being responsive to rather than rejecting of demands which might stimulate community activity*;
- *being prepared to take a lead or pro-active role in getting a new development going*;
- *withdrawing from leadership roles* – so that people from the community can take them on;
- *making links between organisations*;
- *making links between welfare needs and general community organisations* – so as to increase the range of support in the community for caring needs and reduce isolation and stigmatisation.

As with linking work, community development work requires a sense of strategy. One fundamental is to help develop organisational bases (Payne, 1986a, pp. 87–98) which give strength and consistency to possible developments, by bringing people together, helping to identify a suitable structure and organisation for the activities they want to do, and helping to identify resources that they can use.

It can be helpful to start from the knowledge of what existing services and resources are available and develop from these. Increasing resources to and fully extending existing services, known to be helpful already, may be the most effective way of developing new provision. It allows workers in new areas or organisations to have contact with and to be trained alongside people already providing the service, and managers to have a model on which they can base their own developments. Service users, carers and people in the community can see the service running and see how and in what ways it can be effective in meeting their needs.

One area of provision, not so far discussed, is the role of volunteer services. These offer individuals who 'through their own free will spend time, unpaid . . . in doing something that aims to benefit someone other than his or her immediate family.' (slightly adapted from Presland, 1990). They either do this as individuals, or through organised groups which seek to promote volunteer involvement in providing services. Surveys (Davis Smith, 1992) show that between a quarter and a half of the adult population provide voluntary services in this way, although regular providers are less common. Volunteers are most likely to be employed in a middle-class job, but this finding reflects the fact that working-class and unemployed people may 'volunteer' in different ways, such as by being involved in community or self-help organisations which do not fit the individualistic definition given above. Such involvement can offer greater participation and control of the direction of what they do than just volunteering individually (Rochester, 1992). The same may apply to people from minority ethnic communities, who can be encouraged to volunteer as a contribution to community care services if they are specifically targeted and made to feel wanted, and their needs and motivations are provided for (Obaze, 1992). People volunteer for a variety of motives, some of which may be altruistic or as a result of religious beliefs, while some may have instrumental purposes, such as getting to know a new area, or gaining experience which will help improve career or job prospects (Leat, 1983; Sherrott, 1983).

If care managers are to make use of volunteers, whether individuals or those from an organised service, Presland (1990) argues that careful attention must be paid to:

- matching the motivations of the particular volunteer with the needs of the person being helped;
- paying careful attention to the volunteer–client relationship, so that it offers social and personal benefits to both;
- the volunteers' independence, so that they are free to decide what they can and want to provide, and do not feel exploited by a service-providing agency – this may be particularly important where the provider is a statutory or private sector organisation, where there may be fears of replacing public sector jobs or supportive private profit;
- helping volunteers to be responsive to clients' needs; their individualistic involvement and potential commitment can be an important characteristic of their advantages as part of a package of services.

Many volunteers offer practical help such as shopping and making a meal for a disabled or older person. Befriending, thus providing useful social contact, is also frequently arranged. Volunteer services can be more complex, including advocacy (Willis, 1992), or education. Service users (for example, people recovering from a mental illness, or someone with disabilities) may well value making a contribution to the community by volunteering, and this can be considered as part of a package as an element of leisure, or personal, or social or educational development.

The difficult issues about volunteering and community care are explored by Heginbotham (1990). He argues that in spite of the individual benefits of volunteering, and its long history, the 'new right' view of volunteering is that it is the only true expression of welfare. If this assumption is followed to its logical conclusion, all collective provision for welfare is considered to be without justification. Privatisation of welfare to that extent involves the removal of the rights of citizens to collective provision for care, deriving from their citizenship. Thus, we have to be careful in promoting the personal advantages of volunteering not to progress towards a view which negates the value of consistent, collective provision for welfare.

Putting it all together

Throughout Chapters 5 and 6, we have been examining various potential parts of a care plan, and the skills involved in implementing those parts. Completing this process takes us back to our starting point. The beginning of Chapter 5 was concerned with the interpersonal process of agreeing the plan; here we must be concerned with the interpersonal process of implementing it. As a process, it is a series of events which take place over *time* and which are *connected to each other*. The events involve *people* and *organisations*. Actual, potential and desired connections between these people and organisations must be defined and commitments to the proposed arrangements achieved among these people and organisations. Such commitments will require confirmation, affirmation and consideration, in order to create an exchange. The processes of monitoring and review (see Chapter 8) must be established to check that what has been confirmed, affirmed and for which consideration has been provided are actually operating as intended, and what was intended is actually beneficial.

Implementing a care plan, requires, first, an understanding of the time structure of what is planned. Ideally, an entire care package should not be introduced at once, particularly if it is a complex one. This is unnecessary even in extreme circumstances. For example, in considering discharge from hospital, there must come a point at which the individual is formally discharged. Plans for the care package may be made in advance. Mrs Porteous, for example, had a serious fall while living alone and stayed in the geriatric ward of a local hospital for several weeks. Discharge was planned. She received physiotherapy to make her limbs more mobile on the ward, and visited her home several times, for assessment of various abilities, and to plan the provision of aids and adaptations, which arrived over several subsequent weeks. When she had improved sufficiently, and all the essential aids had arrived, she was discharged, home help and district nursing services resumed and further aids were delivered as they became available.

As another example, Mr Green, a man recovering from very long-term mental illness, was discharged to a group home to join two others already living there; a former resident had died. He received an extensive training programme at the hospital, before the home was identified. Then the community team arranged for introduction to the house, and he spent several weekends, then days there. He was also introduced to the related day centre. It was several months before he was formally discharged and moved all his property.

These examples show that implementation of a plan can be seen as a pathway, in which there are gates along the way, at each of which a new direction is taken. Workers need to identify the gates, and see which workers and organisations are relevant to that change of direction, and what actions are necessary. The client's progress then forms the connection between the different stages of implementing the plan.

As each group of workers and organisations is identified for each gate, agreement about their part in the total picture needs to be made, and the connections between them identified which will be required for the plan to be implemented. These will very often be defined and confirmed by a written agreement, part of the community care system's contracting. However, more than confirmation is required: workers will need to consider motivating the people involved in their commitment to the clients and the plan. A long-standing carer, for example, may have no problems in personal commitment to the client, but may be insecure about whether a complicated plan is going to work, or unsure about how they are going to give up part of a role that they have previously taken themselves. A newly-involved home help, on the other hand, may have a conventional way of working, which may not fit well with the particular needs of the client or wishes of the carer. The worker must gain affirmation from people involved, an enthusiastic participation in the planning and the implementation of it. An important aspect of this is ensuring they take on the responsibility to raise problems and issues as they arise, rather than suffering silently, or over-doing things themselves.

Another important aspect is consideration, using this term in the legal sense, of making sure that people get their rewards for their involvc.. ent. Where this is part of the local authority's contracting system, payments will be required; where the rewards are more personal, reassurance about the importance of people's roles, confirmation of their value, and commitment to staying with them are crucial aspects of helping the implement the plan.

This emphasis on the interpersonal aspects of making a care plan work leads us directly on to the importance of user and carer involvement, and it is to this topic that the next chapter pays attention.

7

Empowerment and Advocacy for Users' Interests

The professional and policy context

Community care policy fosters clients' choice as an important part of the service. This is partly for political reasons, since the government's commitment to a market system requires potential consumers to have enough information to make informed decisions about their requirements. Markets only succeed in advancing competition if there are alternatives to choose from, and choice is only possible if clients know about possible alternatives. In addition to this, professional opinion has been developing a concern for user participation in professional decisions, and theory and methodology about empowerment and advocacy.

Post-Griffiths community care policy contains three aspects which potentially promote users' choices and empowerment:

- *communication* about the services available in general and in each local authority area;
- *an empowering approach* in the work of the social workers and others who implement care management and provide services (see Chapter 6) including facilities for making complaints and having representation in decision-making;
- *the development of advocacy services* on behalf of users.

Following this introductory contextual discussion, this chapter contains a section on each of these aspects of policy and practice.

Official guidance

Community care policy recognises similar requirements. The *NHS &CCA, 1990*, for example, requires local authorities to publish their community care plans and complaints procedures (Section 46, 52 (Scotland); 50, 52 (Scotland) respectively), and the policy guidance (DoH, 1990, pp. 16, 19, 34) sets out a variety of information that local authorities should publish. This is dealt with more extensively in both the practice and management guidance on care management (SSI/SWSG, 1991a and b, pp. 31–5, 41–2, respectively), because, as we have seen in Chapter 3, the principles of care management assume efforts to screen the population for everyone who is likely to need services, and an essential part of this is to offer widespread information to generate contact with people who might be in need. Guidance on community care planning, examined in the next two chapters, proposes measures like population needs assessment (Price Waterhouse, 1993) to explore the range and quantity of needs which might exist in a local authority area.

The care management practice guidance (SSI/SWSG 1991a, p.33) emphasises the needs-led nature of the service as the crucial basis of the information, and so it seems to want to support the change of approach implied by community care policy by helping the public, and other people who need information to understand the service in a new way. Both the policy guidance and the care management practice guidance concentrates on the public and clients' understanding of assessment procedures in particular, on the assumption that this is what will gain them access to services, and so therefore it is the crucial part of the maze of services that the public must find their way through.

The importance of the publication of information as seen by official eyes was signalled when the SSI published even more detailed guidance on communication with the public (SSI, 1991). This is the first time there has been such an emphasis in British social services policy.

Professional context

However, the official importance given to this whole area reflects the increasing professional concern for these issues. This can be seen in:

- developing social work practice theory;
- the growth of theories of empowerment and advocacy as part of social work;
- increasing interest in clients' rights, participation and consumerism as an aspect of social work practice;
- the transfer of ideas of advocacy, citizen advocacy and self-advocacy from areas of practice close to social work; and
- increasing development of complaints procedures and advocacy in similar legislation and practice guidance emanating from the DoH, described above.

To understand the increasing role given to these aspects of practice in post-Griffiths community care policy and practice, we need to examine each of these areas of development in turn.

Clients' rights in social work practice theory

Traditional social work practice theories tend to be 'expert' theories; that is, they assume that the social worker is a professional person who helps the client from a position in which the worker has expertise which he or she conveys to or uses on the client. Finkelstein (1990) argues that this kind of view leads professionals to have a limited view of 'normality' which implies that disabled people are abnormal because they cannot function in the ordinary activities of daily life. Their problem is seen as personal, rather than recognising, for example, that much of the 'social and physical environment' (p. 40) is arranged for those who are 'normal'. He argues that we should see disability as an interaction between people's capacities and the environment we establish. Many long-standing ideas in social work come from psychological or medical-psychiatric theories, such as psychoanalysis (Payne, 1992), behaviour and learning theory and cognitive theory, and these all tend to work from the assumption of expertise.

Assuming such a degree of incapacity in clients is not necessarily true of all such theories, however. Behavioural social work theory, for example, while relying on the technical expertise of the professional, also proposes a degree of openness with clients. Task-centred social work (being developed from 1969 onwards) formalises and extends such an approach within the social work tradition, by stimulating the client's involvement in defining a clear set of problems, and the worker and client sharing in a series of tasks directed explicitly towards resolving the major problem selected for action (Doel and Marsh, 1992). This more explicit form of personal therapy relies on a (sometimes written) 'contract' or agreement about planned action between worker and client. While there is controversy about the extent to which this genuinely liberates clients' participation (since the status of the parties is – sometimes covertly – unequal to start with), it has drawn workers' attention to the importance of gaining clients' commitment to and involvement in treatment aims and the action taken to achieve them.

Since the 1970s, the trend towards assuming greater participation in and control of social work by clients has developed. This was fostered in the first instance by sociological approaches to social work, such as systems or role theory. Because such theories emphasise the importance of the social origins of many of the problems which clients face, they are not so inclined to emphasise clients' personal incapacities, and therefore lead to an assumption of greater equality between worker and client. Radical theories, while they can presume that the worker's appreciation of the social origins of oppression is greater than the clients, emphasise working alongside the client to further social progress even more strongly. Developments of radical ideas, such as feminist therapy, stress shared experience between worker and client forcefully. Further exploration of these and other aspects of social work theories may be found in Payne (1991).

Empowerment and advocacy in social work theory

Two important recent developments in social work theory have further emphasised empowerment and advocacy theory. Philp (1979), in a discussion of the role of social work, notes how an essential part of all social work is interpreting people who are 'outsiders' in society to those who are in powerful positions. In the late 1970s and 1980s, theories of practice specifically directed towards this aspect of social work developed, including Solomon's (1976) 'black empowerment', advocacy theories based on the radical work of Freire (1972) in Latin America, such as that of Rose and Black (1985) working with people being discharged from psychiatric hospitals in the USA.

In a recent formulation of these ideas, Rees (1991) identifies five aspects which define empowerment theory.

- *Biography* People's ability to gain power over their surroundings, or their inability to do so, is rooted in their life history, which sets up what Solomon (1976) would call 'blocks' which must be overcome and which also offers experiences which can help understanding of what is happening to us and strengthen our capacity to cope.
- *Power* Empowerment examines direct influence on social situations that we take part in and other dimensions, including power and disempowering circumstances, which are built into society and affect us all.
- *Politics* All uses of power are political, in that they are concerned with gaining power over resources which affect many people's lives.
- *Skills* Skills in interacting with others help people gain power; negotiation, advocacy and assessment and evaluation are crucial to giving people power over their circumstances.
- *Policy and practice are interdependent* Often we separate ideas about practice from the policy which creates the environment within which we practise. Meethan and Thompson (1993), for example, studied the introduction of a multi-disciplinary community care pilot scheme, and identified many conflicts among stakeholders, including politicians, in the development of the scheme. They argue that so many interests have to be accommodated that users' concerns can become excluded.

This brief account of Rees's analysis demonstrates many connections with the approach to community care that I have taken in this book. Resources and power over them are crucial to making a success of community care. I have tried to show that the kinds of indirect practice skills that Rees says are essential to empowerment are important for successful community care practice and, in particular, how the understanding of how practice and policy interact is a key part of community care.

Moxley (1989) regards 'self-direction' by clients as central to American case management, because it is expected by society, can reduce dependence on professionals and services and can help the client to reach higher levels of autonomy in managing his or her affairs. He argues for it on the basis that as a matter of values clients are entitled to as much independence as possible, because if the worker expects independence, this will also colour the expectations of clients; it will provide the basis for developing appropriate skills in the client and because the helping relationship can provide a focus for developing self-direction, will also strengthen the client's capacities.

Marsh and Fisher (1992) propose a 'partnership' approach to social work with clients in a variety of social work settings. This involves:

● only investigating problems with the user's consent;
● only intervening if the user agrees or statutory requirements permit;
● basing intervention on the views of all relevant family members;
● basing interventions on negotiated agreement, not assumptions or conventions;
● offering users the greatest possible choice.

This approach is similar to that discussed by Fiedler (1993), in relation to 'getting results' in community care with disabled people. He proposes that making services more responsive requires a clear sense of *purpose*, including clear shared intentions and targets for both services and user involvement, and a *strategy* to create organisational structures and to develop methods of participation. This project for disabled people focuses on responsive planning systems and varied paths for participation as well as individual empowerment to help people participate.

Clients' rights, participation and consumerism in social work

Practice theory is not the only basis in social work for the importance of client participation, and choice. A significant value base in social work has been the principle of client self-determination. This has developed from early ideas that social work would be more effective if it engaged clients' motivation by encouraging them to participate in decisions within the social work process. Such views of 'therapeutic efficiency' were enhanced to form value position that clients were entitled to (limited, according to Biestek, 1961, p. 103) freedom of action which should be respected by workers. Some took a '*self-realisation*' view (for example, Bartlett, 1970, pp. 65–6) arguing that self-determination helped to achieve the best possible realisation of each individual's potential and therefore an evolutionary growth in society's potential. The *radical* view (for example, Bailey and Brake, 1975) criticised both these positions, arguing that such expressed values were ineffective in a society where most of the people who received social work services were oppressed and disadvantaged by the dominance of economically and politically powerful groups.

Responding to this, a movement for 'client participation' (BASW, 1980) grew up, arguing for social work methodologies and values which actively promoted participation in decisions and actions, rather than a rather vague acceptance of a right to 'self-determination'. This recognised the limitations on self-determination: at least participation meant some influence, even if it was not a determining one. Such views are explicitly based on 'citizenship' (for example, Jordan, 1975; Beresford and Croft, 1993) which proposes that citizens receiving services from public institutions in a democratic society should be entitled to more than distant participation in decisions by exercising their vote, but a more active daily participation in decisions which affect them. Citizenship views (for example, Biehal, 1993) argue that individual rights to participation are important as well as more effective in developing equality and social justice than decentralisation and local management advocated by, for example, Hadley and Hatch (1981) and in community social work methods.

Participation as a citizen is, however, different from participation as a 'consumer'. The client participation movement is related to the application of ideas from the wider consumerism movement, which grew up in the 1970s. Consumerism is a movement which responds to 'excessive business power in "buyer-seller" relationships' (Kroll and Stampfl, 1981, p. 97) in the commercial world. Applying such approaches to public services is difficult, because it means one part of government policing another. Also, the problem for consumers of the public services is usually rationing: they want a service which the public authority cannot afford or provide. This requires a *justice model* in which clients can appeal or an advocacy or participation model which forces better information into the decision-making processes of the public authority. A *consumer model* which assumes that a product or service is easily available, but has failed through incompetence or dishonesty is not very relevant where choice is not available, however well informed a client may be. To deal with such situations, where they arise, a complaints procedure can be a useful part of a strategy for empowerment and advocacy by allowing a process of review to begin or to question a decision-making process, but unless citizenship confers rights to service, merely being regarded as a consumer does not offer choice in a constrained public service. Potter (1988) argues that there are four major elements in a consumerist policy

- access
- choice
- information
- representation.

All these are represented to some degree in post-Griffiths community care policy, but McGrath and Grant (1992) argue that active incentives must be offered to draw users and carers into participation, in the same way that incentives have proved necessary to ensure health and social services co-operation.

Another problem with the consumer approach in general and which also applies to consumerism in public services, is that many consumerist strategies can be taken into the service and used to consumers' disadvantage. For example, we have seen how government seeks to use consumer participation in services to restrict professional discretion in 'common-sense' ways. This might mean, for example, that uninformed or prejudiced consumer involvement could disadvantage minority groups (for example, residential care places should be given to local white people before people from minority ethnic communities). 'Common sense' might lead to demands for more expenditure on home care for older people than for mentally ill people. Information on consumer needs in the population can just as easily be used to justify not providing a service to marginal groups, or to inform targeting and rationing policies, by helping to draw criteria of need more tightly.

A further difficulty in including users' views as consumers is that their assumptions and the organisations which they would prefer to offer services to them are excluded by the assumptions and attitudes prevalent in the service. The most obvious example lies in the provision of services to minority ethnic groups. Atkin (1991) argues that we tend to assume that if we understand attitudes among users in minority ethnic communities, we can adapt the nature of our services to their needs. However, it may be that different groups would reject our assumptions about appropriate kinds of service or the organisations that are commonly used to provide services, or would differ in their views about these aspects of provision. Many groups might prefer service-delivery by agencies managed by people from their own communities, for example. This possibility draws attention to the fact that our basic assumptions in organising a service might be alien, not only to minority ethnic groups but many other particular communities as well.

Advocacy in related areas of practice

We focused above on the application of advocacy and empowerment theory within professional activities. A more extensive application of advocacy as a concept has developed within mental health work and a variety of areas close to social services.

The classic example of advocacy is that of the lawyer for a client in a court of law. However, lawyers' professional power and social status often gives them excessive control over what they do, so that only powerful clients, such as large businesses, can control and demand lawyers' adherence to what their clients want. Also, lawyers operate on a fee-for-service basis and charge high fees, so that their services, except where legal aid is relevant, are mostly unavailable to disadvantaged users of the social services. This means that using the law and legal advocacy skills is not possible in any but very controversial or important community care cases.

Lawyers' advocacy is in an individual matter, on behalf of a person or corporate body. Bull (1982) and Rees (1991) usefully distinguish 'cause' advocacy from 'case' advocacy. Cause advocacy is arguing for the reform of a system. Bull thinks the two can be related. Arguing for a cause can be improved by getting close knowledge of relevant cases and so being in touch with all the details. Arguing for a cause resolves many individual cases of difficulty. Patti (1971, p. 537) argues that, in similar fashion workers should take responsibility for internal advocacy, arguing for change within their agencies for the benefit of clients. There has been debate about the extent to which workers should concentrate on arguing to change to a general situation rather than dealing with individual problems. The Ad Hoc Committee on Advocacy (1969) argued that working at a general level benefits more clients in the long run, but Gilbert and Specht (1976) argue that the principle should be 'first, do no harm' to and concentrate on the needs of the individuals with whom a worker is presented. Cause advocacy should be added to that.

The problem with professional advocacy of this kind is that if an advocate takes on a case, he or she can remove responsibility for acting for themselves from the client; this can be to their future disadvantage. Also, professional, managerial or time pressures on workers may cause them to avoid pushing advocacy fully on behalf of clients, and pushing for one case may disadvantage another, or another group. Another difficulty may be that workers have their own interests and concerns in a service and cannot present the client's views fully, or the client's views conflict with their own position. For example, I was involved with advocacy on behalf of a group in a residential care home that was being closed down. The residents claimed that they had not been consulted about the closure. The (extremely caring) managers said that they had no choice, because part of the building was unsafe, and they did not want to worry residents until they found a resolution. The residents felt that they could have contributed to the solution and prepared themselves for a necessary move, and I felt that such advance preparation would have helped the residents settle quicker when they did move. In this case, the managers, out of the best of intentions, prevented the residents from having a say in matters which affected them and treated them (courteously and considerately) as less than responsible for their own lives. Their concern for efficiency and the best solution ignored the importance of involvement.

For this reason, a variety of different advocacy approaches have grown up.

- *Citizen advocacy* works on a one-to-one basis, where volunteers befriend and get to know the views of someone who cannot speak for themselves because of physical or learning disability, and represent their views where needed, for example, at case conferences. The advantages of this are economy and on-going relationships which enable the advocate to gain a close acquaintance over time with the client's views and progress. The problem is that, unless carefully handled, such advocacy can become little more than a volunteer counselling relationship, and the client is less likely to gain skills for representing themselves.
- *Self-advocacy* is designed to deal with some of the problems of professional and citizen advocacy, by providing training and group support to help people learn the skills and gain the emotional

strength to advocate for themselves. The problem with this is that problems can be too complex and difficult, and the skills of the people involved inadequate to the task of dealing with very complex bureaucracies such as that associated with community care.

- *Group advocacy* tries to deal with some of these problems, by bringing together a group of people with similar interests, so that they operate as a group to represent their shared interests. The problems with this are that interests may not all be shared, so some needs may not be met, and that the complexities of dealing with group process may lead to problems (for example, some people may dominate inappropriately). It can also produce leading members, who then feel a lot of personal pressure, and who can feel an unreasonable sense of failure, whereas a professional advocate would be less pressurised by such feelings.

It may be useful to combine a number of these features. Self-advocacy supported by a strong group or self-help organisation, with professional help, training and support and a professional advocate to call in when more complex situations arise, can combine the benefits of all these models of advocacy. Considerable development in the advocacy field has led to a much more explicit and demanding conceptualisation of the possibilities, and this enables us to look critically at what community care policy offers in this field.

Communication with community care users

Following its policy for user involvement, the DoH has pursued two avenues of development. The first is to encourage SSDs to present the changes in policy very widely, clearly and effectively to users. One aspect of this is the first stage of care management which, we noted in Chapter 3, starts from providing information about services to the public. The second, dealt with in the next section, is concerned with encouraging professionals to be more involving as they deal with clients.

The guidance on communication (SSI, 1991c) confirms that information should be produced for users about

- policies and procedures

- needs that they can and will meet
- services available
- ways of gaining access to services.

It emphasises the importance of clarity about what is intended, without which it is impossible to communicate about it, and wide consultation. Clarity should include certainty about values and principles of the intended services. Information should take account of people with difficulties in reading due to disability or differences in culture or language, and the guidance emphasises the importance of avoiding jargon. A survey of 100 users showed that none understood 'network' and few understood 'gender', 'criteria' and 'equitable manner'. Some thought that 'voluntary agency' meant 'people with no experience', 'sensitive' meant 'tender and sore' and 'agencies' meant 'second-hand clothes shop'. This shows how routine social services terms can lead to confusion for clients. The guidance focuses strongly on referral, assessment and review (that is, monitoring) procedures, rather than entitlements to service, which might be difficult to describe, and might also commit the agency to more than it would want to admit to.

A subsequent survey of achievements in this area (KPMG Peat Marwick, 1993) looked at achievements in 12 local authorities. Publicity material had been made available in most, but had little effect on users, who were still poorly informed about assessment and charging. SSDs had not consulted user and carer groups about information, and often did not have an information strategy or effective information systems. As a result, leaflets went out of date or were not widely available. Another problem was that most users and carers approached people that they knew within the services, and these workers were ill-informed, because the department did not consider them to be appropriate information providers. So home helps or day care staff did not have or were wrong about information, because the departments regarded the responsibility of providing information as residing in offices or with social workers.

Information provision in offices and for social workers, therefore, needs efficient organisation, with a comprehensive stock of leaflets, and a system for ordering more when they are running low (rather than running out). Social workers need to include in their work the provision of documents for clients and carers. It is a professional responsibility to make departments aware of inadequacies in the range of leaflets available, and to suggest improvements in language and design. As well as carers and users, workers who can give feedback on how leaflets are used and responses from clients should be involved in planning and design.

Departments should have a much wider concern for the range of staff who might come into contact with members of the public. Extensive training on the values, basic provision and procedures in the service will be required for all workers. Knowledge of the information system, and a recognition among managers and workers that all staff have responsibilities for disseminating information to clients are required.

Users and their carers are supposed to be involved in the planning and organisation of services. Hoyes and Taylor (1993) reported a preliminary study of experiences of users' and carers' organisations in four local authorities about involvement in this way. Local authorities had used mainly established networks of contacts in larger voluntary organisations, rather than smaller and less formal user groups. Those involved felt that decisions had been taken, rather than that they were really responsive to participation. Training and facilitation of people who have little experience of such participation may be important, and a useful role that social workers can play. Some people from the community were opposed to provision from the independent sector, because it was less certain, and there was doubt that resources would be available to meet the promise of flexible care management.

Empowerment as part of social work in community care

Examining the process of care management earlier in this book, we have seen the emphasis given to involving users and carers in decisions and social work activities. Involvement, advocacy and empowerment are growing theoretical and ethical strengths in social work practice. Why, then, is it that developing user involvement is seen as such a difficult and important issue? One perspective on this issue is given by the Audit Commission (1992a) which argues that local authorities need a new culture. They are said to have difficulty in accepting a mixed economy of care, preferring to manage services themselves; think that we should not limit services to the most dependent, and therefore do not introduce adequate priority systems;

reject separation of purchasing and providing functions, seeing it as privatisation; and have an inflexible centralised operating style which does not give enough flexibility to staff and is poor at setting clear goals and values and obtaining staff commitment to them. This account emphasises the process of introducing the government's preferred management strategy, and lays the problems at the door of local government.

Stevenson and Parsloe (1993), reviewing this issue, argue that many workers do not experience their organisations as empowering. Workers will be free to be more empowering as they feel a shared responsibility and independence in carrying out their work. Also, empowering managers offer a model of good practice to workers; bureaucrats do not. Managers, in Stevenson and Parsloe's view, should have and convey a clear concept of how they expect workers to behave and what attitudes they should display. Clarity about systems, responsibilities and legal powers and responsibilities also helps. On the other hand, one study of social and health workers (Dalley, 1989) shows that managers can be less hostile to clients than direct workers because they are not pressurised by them every day. Workers need to have considerable space to make decisions and work in their own way, but in some areas need to be clear that they are working to legal or administrative requirements. This feature of social work practice requires a balanced approach to management which is hard to maintain. Flexibility and space is often limited in the wrong places by procedural correctness, and yet workers lack clarity where it ought to exist. Stevenson and Parsloe recommend (p. 11) an openness to debate and disagreement and to negotiate rather than seek to win arguments. This recommendation for good management is sometimes inconsistent with the hierarchical systems and procedural correctness which infect local government. Brokerage systems (see Chapter 3) of care management, rather than, or as an adjunct to, social care entrepreneurship models of care of management may offer a less hierarchical, more sharing approach to community care practice.

Another reason for the concern about workers' capacity to operate in a way which empowers users and carers is the traditional individualistic, psychological assumptions of social work theory and practice. We saw at the beginning of this chapter that these often assume that social work deals with abnormality rather than interactions between a society which does not encourage difference and those who are different. Stevenson and Parsloe (p. 22) point to one of the factors that strengthens such a view, that social workers often in reality deal with people's increasing dependence, and this seems inconsistent with empowerment. However, people who are elderly or suffer from learning difficulties may need for their own peace of mind and that of people around them to hand over some practical responsibilities. One of the tasks of the worker is to seek out responsibilities which can be empowering and which they are able to accept, and help them to retain responsibilities which are emotionally important to them, shedding those which they are relieved to lose. One aspect of this, as we saw in Chapter 5, is balancing risk of dangerous outcomes against opportunities for empowerment and balancing the anxiety of carers and perhaps other officials against clients' needs for independence and empowerment.

Stevenson and Parsloe (1993) present a formulation of empowering methods of working within community care:

- a clear value and policy framework, based on clients setting agendas for work and priorities;
- effective methods of practice which include a variety of communication methods, including concentration on non-verbal communication; careful pacing of the work, so that clients do not have to take on too much at once, and the worker's effort is not dissipated in too many directions; a negotiation approach (see Chapter 5) which enables needs and services to be 'worked out' jointly rather than presented intact to a client; the inclusion of effective 'counselling' proposed in Chapter 5 as the 'glue' of delivering a package of services, and effective networking and indirect work (see Chapter 6).

Solomon (1989) emphasises the importance of people recognising that

- although not responsible for causing problems, clients have responsibility for resolving them;
- workers have expertise to contribute to help with that responsibility;
- clients and helpers work as peers, not as professional and client;
- relationships with other social institutions may affect the problem, and need to be tackled; and

● the social system is not impenetrable, but is made up of many small parts which can be influenced and changed.

Several writers (for example, Parsloe, 1986; Adams, 1990; Rees, 1991) argue the importance of helping clients to understand the political nature of their personal problems, and Adams (p. 125) emphasises the importance of being prepared to transfer resources, rather than delegating them with the worker retaining control. Moxley (1989) argues that the crucial features of the helping role which will empower clients in American case management are:

● accepting and respecting the client
● open and responsive communication with the client
● using and sticking to contracts.

Raiff and Shore (1993, pp. 79–84), in making similar points, also suggest that workers should try to develop clients' and carers' skills in linking and negotiating, since this develops their capacity for equal participation in the community care system.

Complaints and representative machinery

The possibility of clients of SSDs making complaints, has a long history. In central and local government, MPs and councillors investigate complaints and the 'ombudsmen' (Parliamentary and Local Government Commissioners) have been a final recourse for serious complaints. There are also specialist means of complaints, such as the role of the Mental Health Act Commission in overseeing compulsory admissions to mental hospital and giving guidance on mental health services generally through its Code of Practice (DoH/Welsh Office, 1993). Sometimes, it is possible for clients to seek judicial review of official decisions in the courts, or to raise problems through court cases in child care matters and administrative procedures such as compulsory admissions in mental health and Mental Health Review Tribunals.

In the 1980s, there has been greater interest in developing complaints procedures. This has two purposes: one aims to improve the management of agencies by helping to identify and resolve problems; the second is to provide clients with formal mechanisms for redress where they are dissatisfied with decisions or actions of SSD staff. Complaints procedures have been incorporated into child care legislation (Section 26(3), *Children Act, 1989*), and into the *NHS&CCA, 1990* (Section 50 inserts a new Section 7B into the *Local Authority Social Services Act, 1970*, providing for the Secretary of State to make directions on complaints procedures, which process incorporates complaints under the *Disabled Persons (Services, Consultation and Representation) Act, 1986*. As a result of directions, complaints procedures have been in place since April 1991. According to the *Policy Guidance* (DoH, 1990), which presses this issue strongly, procedures must enable people to make complaints, ensure that these are acted on, resolve them quickly and at a low level in the organisation, allow people to challenge decisions to refuse a service, provide for independent review of defined categories of complaint and provide means for managers to monitor performance. Complaints which are not dealt with adequately might lead to complainants seeking judicial review of the local authority's decision and procedures (Gordon, 1993, pp. 54–65).

Practice Guidance is available on how to implement complaints procedures (SSI, 1991a), and an advice booklet for front-line staff such as receptionists who are likely to receive people making complaints (SSI, 1991b). This establishes a process by which there is a 'senior officer' in the SSD responsible for ensuring that complaints are dealt with, and a 'designated complaints officer' (DCO) who deals with all day-to-day matters concerning complaints. There should be an informal, problem-solving stage, and if the matter is not dealt with successfully there, it should be registered. An investigator is appointed, who reports to the DCO, giving the manager of the service a chance to respond to the report. The Department then considers what action it will take. After this, dissatisfied complainants may take the matter to a review by members of the Council. Training for those directly involved, and information for staff and service users, should be available.

Two issues arise for practitioners. The first is how they react themselves when receiving complaints or being complained about. Although this is unpleasant and stressful, workers need to encourage users by their positive attitude in exercising their rights and questioning decisions. Such a questioning attitude is an indication of people actively participating in decisions and care provision, and is to be welcomed. The second issue for practitioners lies in the extent to which they encourage users to make complaints and use the systems available to them. Obviously, it is not to a user's advantage to be seen as difficult, nobody wants to stimulate complaints about themselves and users should not be manipulated to gain advantage for a worker or group of workers in the battle for resources and internal political advantage. However, complaining or seeking a review of a decision can be a useful strategy for a user who does not receive an appropriate service as a result of a care manager's assessment. Workers may, therefore, want to help users make complaints, refer them to advocacy groups who can help them, or help in setting up advocacy groups.

Advocacy as part of community care

The essential difference between advocacy and, say, negotiation on a client's behalf, is that advocacy occurs in a situation in which there is opposition. Either a decision has been made which the client considers unfavourable or action has been taken which they are dissatisfied with. The client's feelings about what had happened (or not happened) to him or her are therefore one crucial element. Another important factor is the process that needs to be followed to resolve the clients feelings. If this is oppositional, we are dealing with advocacy, but it helps our humanity to see ourselves as opposing what has gone wrong, rather than other people. In particular, we should avoid setting client against client or client against colleague. It is advocacy, for example, if the worker is arguing the client's case against others in an allocation meeting for scarce resources: the opposition here is not between clients, but against shortage of resources. It is advocacy if the worker supports a client through a complaint procedure: the opposition is not someone who is wrong, but an experience which must be questioned.

It is important to distinguish between advocacy schemes which offer advocacy on behalf of clients, to enable them, for example, to use complaints procedures effectively, and advocacy on behalf of clients by workers as part of their social work role. Providing independent advocacy schemes is an application of the community social work skills of setting up and supporting groups, and linking skills in dealing with independent groups effectively. Although professional support – both practical help and principled support for the idea that such advocacy should be available – is needed to establish such groups, they are properly independent of the main providing agencies. As with self-help groups, a specialised centre or co-ordinating group for local advocacy groups may benefit them, and might be an appropriate function of a local council for voluntary service or other voluntary sector co-ordinating body.

Within service-providing organisations, a 'culture of advocacy' (Dalrymple, 1993) must be built up which accepts the role that advocacy on behalf of clients can play. Otherwise, workers can be unreasonably resistant to suggestions or demands made by clients through advocacy. It is easy to be offended when there is criticism of decisions when the worker has made an effort to develop commitment to effective and caring management. Even so, professional opinion may not fit what the client wants. Advocacy will struggle and may fail, if professional workers do not respond to it by listening carefully, explaining and justifying their actions, and changing their mind and policies when they are shown to be unsatisfactory to clients. Another crucial professional role in advocacy schemes is supporting them by providing training and help in developing the skills of negotiation and communication in clients, carers and advocates.

Advocacy also arises as part of ordinary professional roles. One aspect of this may be that every action of a social worker in creating and implementing a package of services means interpreting the client's needs and conveying them to providers of the service. So the care manager is inevitably advocating, in the sense of interpreting and responding to the client's wishes. In many cases, the worker will also have a central role in fighting for the client's interests within the agency or in a related agency. Even so, it is important to recognise that sometimes what the worker interprets as the client's best interest may not be the preferred course of the client. Having advocated as a professional, then, the worker may face an independent client's advocate or the client or carer themselves presenting a case against what has been achieved.

Advocacy also interacts with other procedures within agencies. Most important is the disciplinary and grievance procedures, since a complaint sometimes triggers action against an employee by the employer, and complaints by a member of staff. Usually, these procedures are much more powerful in agencies than client complaints procedures or advocacy schemes, and also they have a much higher standard of evidence and formality of procedure. As a result, a client can become mixed up, sometimes as a witness, with such procedures, to find that the worker is not disciplined or their grievance is accepted, and the complaint is dismissed without their own feelings and experiences being fully explored. In one case, for example, the client made a complaint about rudeness and aggression by the worker. This was subjected to a semi-judicial procedure, with the worker represented by his trade union. Because of this, the worker was instructed by his representatives not to acknowledge the client's feelings, since this would have been an admission of guilt. The disciplinary procedures found in favour of the worker, and the local authority therefore rejected the client's complaint, and insisted that since the worker had been found 'not guilty' the client must accept him back as her main carer. If this happens, the client is very often left without support, and it is impossible for staff to acknowledge their feeling of having been wronged and how bad they feel. A simple 'I'm sorry you've had a bad time' seems impossible to offer. Workers in this situation, and advocates, need to respect clients' feelings, acknowledge and do something about the fact that even the procedure can feel like a violent abuse and think carefully about their future care even if the complaint is unsuccessful.

Turning now to professional advocacy on behalf of clients, it is useful to explore practice opportunities in four phases within the process:

● *exploration* – where clients' experiences and feelings about them, and in particular their wishes about what should happen can be identified;
● *preparation* – where clients' wishes can be expressed within the agency, ways of taking them up explored and if necessary, a formal case for a complaint or other procedure prepared;
● *advocacy* – where clients' wishes are pressed within the agency; and
● *termination* – where the aftermath of the resolution and clients' feelings about it are dealt with. As with clients who are using advocacy schemes, this phase is easy to forget, but very important if clients are to respect the process which has taken place and move forward positively again.

In the exploration phase, workers should explore the details of the

incident which has led to a complaint or bad feeling. Often, one
incident which seems unexceptional means that the worker must focus
on a longer period of difficulties which has built up feelings about
the situation which are stronger than the present incident can justify.

The resolution that the clients want is important. Where an apology is the desired outcome, the worker would act differently from
where compensation or a change in the service provided is sought.
There are fundamentally six levels of resolution that might be achieved,
and several might be sought in any one situation:

- *compensation* – by apology or financial recompense;
- *reinstatement* – by establishing or re-establishing the client's
  desired outcome;
- *reconsideration* – by establishing that new information or argument allows a charge in the decision;
- *rule-bending* – by establishing that the rules might be applied
  in different way;
- *exception* – by establishing that this particular client should be
  excepted from the rules or standard procedures;
- *policy-change* – by establishing that the way policy is applied
  or the policy itself should be changed.

The reality of the difficulty must be explored. For example, a disabled man had difficulty with a claim for a benefit which he thought
had been rejected. In reality, the Benefits Agency had asked for a
form to be completed, and the client had missed the point of this.
In another case, a worker asked me for help in gaining a place for
a man with difficult mental health problems in residential care in
an organisation I worked for, when such a place would have been
freely given (assuming finance was available). Sometimes, people
ask for slightly the wrong thing and are not helped to find the right
alternative. At other times a simple negotiation is enough to resolve
the problem. It does not help a worker's reputation or the needs of
their client to blow a situation up into unnecessary conflict.

In the preparation phase, workers should explore the various alternative procedures that might offer solutions, and agree with their client which is most appropriate. This will generally be the simplest
one to use. They should also agree on the part which the client
should play. If possible, this should be significant; if not, it should
be clear. Sometimes, for example, the worker must go to an internal

meeting to argue the client's case for resources. Even though the client cannot go, their participation might be in preparing the case and arguments and in receiving a report on the result. To strengthen the client's role and skills, it is important in advocacy to be fairly formal about this. Where the client is able to play a part, some rehearsal and role playing of the situation they will experience may be helpful.

In preparing a case, we start from the basis for the decision or event in dispute.

- *Law or policy?* Some circumstances are forced on clients and workers by legal requirements. Is this really true in this case, or is it just a policy that the agency has? If so, can a case be made for an exception?
- *Interpretation?* Whether it is law or policy, has it been interpreted correctly or as intended? Is there an alternative interpretation which can be argued for? Was all the information available and given its proper weight?
- *Fair?* Even where it is interpreted correctly, is it fair? Is there a case for an alternative being more fair to the client? Do we need to focus on fairness for the client rather than someone else?
- *Discretion?* If everything has been done correctly and fairly, but the client's feelings are hurt, is there discretion to take some action to resolve it?
- *The argument?* If the facts and interpretation are right, has the case been argued logically? Do the regulations used really apply to this client's situation, or has someone applied a rule of thumb unwisely? Has the person who made the decision the right to do so?

Starting from the client's preferred outcome, these sort of questions allow you to build up a case to present.

In the advocacy phase, the case must now be presented. The way in which the advocate and client (if present) appear to the panel or individual making a decision is important. Truculence and aggression should be avoided, as also should any challenge to the panel or individual's personal self-image. Ethically, I believe it is also important, as suggested above, to avoid setting client or worker against each other. It is better to set client against resources or decisions, rather than people.

Some useful approaches are as follows.

● *Order of presentation* A strong case for the client and his or her view might come first, with the arguments in favour strongly itemised. Points against should be acknowledged and then each refuted as strongly as possible. Areas of discretion or possible resolution should be pointed out, and suggestions made.
● *Evidence* This needs a clear structure, and if possible too much evidence or repetitive points should be avoided. Documents, especially official ones, often have more credibility than personal evidence, especially from stigmatised people. Too much emotion should be avoided, but feelings and attitudes should be clearly presented and, if possible, explained. If possible, evidence should be vivid: a description of the daily pattern of life or the dangers that they face can help to convince people to act, whereas a 'professionalised' assessment can seem just like any other.

The final phase involves telling the client the outcome: this may come officially, but it may need to be interpreted. The client's feelings (for example, of anger, frustration, or guilt at making things difficult for others, or elation) need to be explored. There should be a forward-looking 'what do we do now?' approach.

In the last four chapters, we have been exploring practice with clients and users of services and their carers. Of course, this focus is not entirely at an end, since clients need to be involved in mechanisms for accountability and policy development which are the focus of the next two chapters. All of the more general systems in community care should be needs-led, and therefore should place clients and users at the centre of what they do. Complaints and information systems, for example, are a crucial part of the accountability mechanisms in community care. It is to these issues, then, that we now move on.

8

Accountability and Effectiveness in Community Care

Accountability issues in community care policy

Community care raises a number of issues about accountability. In this chapter, we shall look at the ways in which post-Griffiths policy tries to deal with these accountability issues, and the consequences for practice. For practitioners, the policy creates multiple and possibly conflicting responsibilities. It seeks to enforce financial limitations and government management philosophies in a context where responsibility to service users' and carers' choice is also being promoted. Workers will feel a responsibility to both sides, and their demands are often in tension. Care management places a responsibility to assess needs and treat these as a priority, while imposing financial limitations on meeting those assessed needs. Different services and professions are also making their own assessments and conflicts between those assessments will have to be worked out.

The changes which have most effect on accountability are as follows.

● *The mixed economy of welfare* This assumes that, rather than the convention of management accountability within one public authority for the quality and availability of a service, a variety of providers will be involved in planning and in offering services. How and to whom will they be accountable for their contribution to planning and to the service? The local authority is responsible for planning, but also for ensuring the participation

198

of service providers in planning, which implies that the authority is accountable to the providers for ensuring their participation. How does the authority decide between potentially equal
providers, when they are entitled to involvement, and how is it
accountable to participants in planning? The basic methods for
accountability by which post-Griffiths policy tries to deal with
these issues are *joint planning* and *contracting*.

- *Care management*   This assumes that one person or service will
  carry out an assessment, and other services will be offered in
  accordance with an individually-tailored care plan by other providers. How do care managers get other providers to offer services according to the care plan, and how do they ensure the
  quality and appropriateness of that provision? Post-Griffiths policy
  tries to deal with these issues by the *purchaser–provider split*,
  delegated budgeting and *implementation monitoring*.

- *User participation*   This assumes that the package provided
  through care management responds to the wishes of the user,
  and that the needs of users or political users affect the community care plan for the area. The ways in which post-Griffiths
  policy tries to deal with these issues involve *user participation
  in care management decisions*, and *information collection and
  feedback* in community care planning. These two aspects of accountability are dealt with in Chapters 7 and 9, respectively.

In addition to these changes in arrangements for accountability at
the local level, the government's 'management approach' means that,
in community care as with other areas of policy, accountability at
central government level is also changing. This is a context of which
practitioners need to be aware of. The system is becoming more
centralised in the sense that central government is taking more responsibility than, say, ten years ago for setting limits within which
policy is implemented. Local authorities are not just left to get on
with implementation. They must comply with the system set up by
central government. For example, the requirement that a high proportion of provision must be in the independent sector limits their
freedom of action. A further pressure is the stream of monitoring
reports and advice and involvement from the SSI. The mixed economy
of care means that groups of private and voluntary providers are
encouraged to become established. The mere fact of their existence
means that local authorities must take notice of and change to take

account of their contribution. Also, the community care planning process enfranchises such groups, giving them a place in local planning and policy-making. On the other hand, increasing complexity means that it is easier for the different parts of it to react in ways that central government would be unable to control. Since private and voluntary sector agencies are providing much of the service, through a series of local agreements, the overall pattern may come to vary widely.

Each area of policy and practice where accountability issues arise fits into a process of mutual accountability between services planners, providers, care managers, and users. If we look again at Figure 2.1 (p. 45), we can see some features of this pattern of accountability: few lines of management accountability exist; practitioners and managers can usefully understand non-managerial relationships between organisations; mutual influence is exercised in purchasing, feedback and provision relationships which were unusual in the previous pattern of government service.

The aim of this chapter is to understand effective work within such relationships. We shall need new ways of evaluating effectiveness and influencing quality in accordance with evaluations. A structure for this is provided within the systems for mutual accountability discussed above, but practitioners will need methods for ensuring quality provision within theire social work practice. The agency structure for quality assurance and enhancement is through *regulation and inspection of provision* and *conditions within contracts*. These, and quality monitoring and evaluation, are the focus of the next part of the chapter. In the following section, the focus moves to *implementation monitoring* within care management, the mechanism by which the individual service provided to users and carers is appraised.

Contracts, regulation and inspection

In many fields of work, local authorities are reducing their role in providing services directly and are entering into contractual relationships with other providers. This does not mean that they give up all responsibility or interests in a particular aspect of their work. Brooke (1989) argues that in this system of government it is the duty of the local authority to become 'enabling' of many of the activities which go on in their area. An authority's power and responsibilities, he argues, require it to interact with related agencies.

Also, councils feel a general responsibility for their whole area and may have goals which they want to press on others. If something goes wrong, the buck often stops with the local authority even where it may be only one participant, and if things need co-ordinating in their area, this often falls to the local authority. Politicians' needs for publicity and involvement may lead to a local authority becoming involved in matters outside its direct responsibilities, and it may be seen as a watchdog for consumers on many matters not strictly within its purview. For all these reasons, Brooke (1989, pp. 12–14), argues, local authorities may become involved in an enabling role. As well as this, in community care they have direct responsibilities to play a lead role in co-ordination and planning. Until recently, they had a leading position as providers, and this continues in many areas for many client groups.

There are a variety of potential relationships between a local authority and others, which Brooke (1989, pp. 11 *et passim*) identifies:

- *control* – putting work out to contract;
- *partial control* – being involved in management or providing part of the service;
- *partnership* – working with another agency to provide a service;
- *part-ownership* – being one of several members of a body which manages a service;
- *purchasing* – influencing the nature of a service by its buying policies;
- *support* – giving financial and practical aid and advice to another agency providing a service;
- *regulation* – regulating and perhaps inspecting services provided by others; and
- *influence* – using its central role in the area to influence how a service is provided.

Each of these types of relationship can be present within the community care system. Sometimes they may be mixed up together: for example, local authorities will be influencing the service given by private care providers (and being influenced in return). As well as this, they will be the major purchaser of such care, and, separately, will be inspecting and registering the provision. There is sometimes controversy about how much regulation and inspection also involves advice and support, but probably several of these processes will involve giving advice and support to private providers.

In an extensive critique of the concept of 'contract' within public services, Harden (1992) argues that there are few differences between the legal concept of contract between individuals and corporate bodies and the legal aspects of contracting with public bodies. However, the idea of contract is 'pregnant with social, economic and political significance' (Harden, 1992, p. 1). It implies freedom to decide who to contract with on the part of the consumer, and a binding requirement to provide service on the part of the provider. However, in reality, these are limited by the power to control the nature of the contract, on the part of the provider, and difficulties in enforcing the consumer's requirements.

Legal powers to enforce standards of provision are complicated in arrangements such as those made by the *NHS&CCA, 1990* by the complicated legal relationships between the consumer and

- a public body providing the service directly;
- a private or voluntary sector organisation with a legal duty to provide the service;
- a service provider with a contract with a public body for providing a service;
- the public body which has contracted with another agency, whether public, private or voluntary, to provide the service; and
- the legal relationship between the public body and the provider.

In most cases, legal responsibility is not clear, and there is no enforceable responsibility to provide services in any particular way, or at all. We have seen how the official guidance about care management and assessment seeks to avoid responsibility for clear statements about levels of provision, and to write financial constraints into arrangements. None the less, there are legally enforceable requirements to carry out assessments, and to respond to them if needs are identified, giving decisions in writing and carrying out financial assessments (Gordon, 1993). How local authorities and providers do their work is also likely to be tested through judicial review in the future (Gordon, 1993).

Harden (1992, pp. 14–17, 42–3) explores the NHS internal market arrangements, which are similar to those made under the community care legislation. He suggests that the absence of a clear contract between patient and health authorities or providers does not enhance the legal rights of patients, or ensure that their preferences are taken into account. Moreover, he argues that the law does not provide a coherent framework for consumers' rights or for the separation of interests where public bodies provide or contract for services. The purchaser or provider's ultimate discretion always remains.

The concept of contract does not provide, therefore, any legal basis for accountability between service users, purchasers or providers. Community care relies, rather, on the commitment of workers and services involved to meeting the requirements that they lay upon themselves to be accountable to consumers and to each other.

Contracts and commissioning

The official guidance to local authorities on contracting (DoH/SSI, 1991) sets out a process in which the local authority moves from its policy goals and aims, to creating a 'service specification', which will include quality systems and standards so that achievement can be measured. Providers may be involved in devising the service specification (para. 3.2.6). The local authority then develops services either 'in-house' or with external providers to create a total service which meets its specifications. At each stage there should be a user and carer perspective as part of the process. In order to make the pattern of service a formal arrangement, the local authority then contracts with particular agencies for their part of the service.

The guidance proposes that there should be eight elements in a service specification, some being more important in a particular instance than others

- *context* – for example, equal opportunities policies, codes of guidance;
- *objectives* – for example, eligibility criteria and how users are consulted;
- *inputs* – for example, budgets, facilities and staffing;
- *process* – for example, methods used;
- *outputs* – 'measurable units of service delivered to clients' (p. 14);
- *outcomes* – the effect on users' wellbeing;
- *quality*; and
- *monitoring*.

Although this sort of process is new to social services, there has been experience of similar processes in local government. The *Local Government Act, 1988*, extended a requirement to put local authority direct labour services out to tender to a wider range of services, mainly of a practical nature, such as cleaning, leisure management and vehicle maintenance (Walsh, 1989); this was extended again to professional services by the *Local Government Act, 1991* (Woolf, 1992). As a result, guidance on organising competitive tenders is available (for example, CIPFA Competition Joint Committee, 1989).

Having made service specifications, local authorities must select service providers. The Policy Guidance (DoH, 1990, p. 41) suggests four alternative approaches to this.

- *Open tendering* The service is advertised, agencies compete to run it. This is only cost-effective (for local authorities and potential providers) for large contracts.
- *Select list tendering* Agencies interested and evaluated as competent are put on a list; a few or all may be offered the chance to tender for particular services. This is most relevant where there are many small providers in competition, epecially where there are variable standards. It is often used for small practical services like plumbing or decorating.
- *Negotiation* Agencies providing or potentially able to provide a service are approached. This can be useful where a particular voluntary or private agency has expertise.
- *Developing new organisations* where none exist or are suitable, or where the market, and competition within it, need enhancing. As we saw in Chapter 5, the 'community care tariff' implies that this will be a low priority for activity where there are other alternatives. However, with many client groups of the social services, provision in a particular area often offers so few choices, that service development, particularly of informal care and support for carers, may be a major aspect of service needs.

A distinction is usually made (by, for example, Flynn and Miller, 1991; Taylor and Vigars, 1993) between 'block' and 'spot' contracts. With block contracts the local authority agrees with providers to receive a specified level of service covering a number of clients. This enables a provider to set up a service, secure in the knowledge that a certain number of clients are going to be referred to justify the setting-up costs. Spot contracts are specific arrangements for an individual client, made where there are many alternative providers, and care managers can be given the budget to make an arrangement, or where there is a specific need (for example, meals on wheels cannot be delivered, so a local cafe is asked to deliver a meal to a specific client) or where a highly specialised service has to be negotiated. The DoH/SSI (1991, p. 20) Guidance identifies these, but argues that spot contracts are only a particular example of 'price by case' contracts in which the cost of each case is defined (for example, a weekly residential charge), but no overall purchase is made. This provides flexibility, but can increase the cost of each case, because the provider must take the financial risk of few cases being referred. A third type of contract identified in the Guidance (DoH/SSI, 1991) is a 'cost and volume' agreement, where a basic level of service is agreed (which allows a provider some certainty) and then additional cases are added on. Here, if there are no alternative providers of a specialised service, the provider might make high charges for additional cases. Sometimes, in all these types of contract, by agreeing a contract for a period, the local authority makes it difficult for alternative suppliers, and so rules out the possibility of changing, if the provider is unsatisfactory.

The local authority may not be the only agency contracting for community care, since health authorities are contracting with agencies for related services. In some areas, for example South Derbyshire (Haggard and Ormiston, 1993), a degree of joint working has been established. Possibilities suggested by these writers include agreeing a joint srategy, requiring providers to work jointly, and seeking feedback from care managers and sevice users on the success of joint working in agencies they are dealing with.

By setting a block contract, the local authority may also rule out other choices for users, who have to accept the provider with the contract. Flynn and Miller (1991, p. 12) argue that authorities should balance the wish to reduce costs by offering large block contracts for long periods (thus reducing the availability of alternatives) and reserving a budget for 'spot' purchases.

Contracting has raised particular issues for voluntary organisations. Many voluntary organisations have been financed by grants, often from local government. Sometimes these have been little more than a contribution to the general running costs of organisations, like a charitable donation, although it may be a gift with conditions attached (Woolf, 1992). Since the 1960s, however, grants to provide particular services have been offered, generally on the basis of a negotiation between the organisation and the authority. The nature of the service has sometimes not been closely specified. In addition to this, voluntary organisations (for example, for residential care) have always provided some services on a price by case basis. During the 1980s, with pressure on local authority budgets, voluntary organisations have used other forms of funding. The Manpower Services Commission and its successors were pre-eminent, offering grants to run a number of training and employment schemes to combat unemployment during the recession of the 1980s. This led many more organisations down the road of receiving grants for providing a service.

Taking on contracts moves a step further. Woolf (1992, p. 9) defines the difference as being that a contract contains an offer (to provide or to pay for a service) and an *unconditional* acceptance of the offer, together with the intention to create a legally binding relationship, where *consideration* (that is, money for services) is exchanged. If voluntary organisations enter such arrangements, they become similar to other independent contractors to the local authority. Their charitable and voluntary status is irrelevant to that particular service.

There may be several problems for a voluntary organisation if it takes on contracts, but there may also be opportunities to achieve service developments (Connor, 1994). Many local voluntary organisations are small, with high fixed costs which the contract may not meet, or the voluntary organisation may be uncompetitive with other larger organisations (Flynn and Miller, 1991, p. 13; DoH, 1993d). Either the staff or the other activities of the organisation are subjected to pressure to use other funds or resources to support the contract as a result. In a small organisation the main purpose may be bent away from general activities towards meeting the terms of the contract. Other work might suffer (for example, campaigning or watchdog functions), because fulfilling a service contract may push the organisation away from it, and there may be a worry that the purchasing local authority will not accept criticism and campaigning about the service from one of its contractors (Hawley, nd, 1992). This leads Flynn and Miller (1991) to suggest that voluntary organisations should get grants for the basic costs of maintaining themselves and for advocacy; in both cases separately from the contracts for service. Sue Lewis (1993), describing the early experience of voluntary organisations, argues that local authorities introducing contracting have been unnecessarily conflictual in their approach, using staff from treasury and legal backgrounds who have little appreciation of the needs of client groups or the sector's provision as a whole. She argues that big companies in the private sector (Marks & Spencer is an often-quoted case) value their supplier network and achieve quality through influence rather than imposition. Community care contracts should be organised on the same basis.

Jane Lewis (1993) suggests that post-Griffiths community care will increasingly redefine the relationship between statutory and voluntary organisations, and formalise it. Reading (nd, 1994) offers a much more comprehensive critique of the role of the voluntary sector in community care. He argues that there is a history within the voluntary sector of being part of a political and moral 'establishment' which may oppress the people that the organisations are there to serve, involving high-status people, for example, to achieve fund-raising or social legitimacy. There is little wide public support or legitimacy for voluntary organisations except at times of national emergency. Although voluntary organisations have the capacity to be innovatory, they must be both insiders and outsiders to the 'establishment' to take on this role. Their role in community care might well bring voluntary organisations more within an oppressive establishment, unless they take on the role of being a broker, as well as an entrepreneur, in the care management process (see Chapter 3). They must also stimulate public debate and evaluation of social objectives in community care services. Reading argues that they must stress the importance of collective responses to social need while not denying the importance of individualisation which is integral to post-Griffiths policy. In this way, the voluntary organisations may be able to develop a less oppressive and individualised moral and political philosophy of community care. He argues that this is essential if voluntary organisations are to maintain their integrity within community care policy.

Grant aid is not, however, excluded from community care arrangements by the official guidance. It (DoH/SSI, 1991, pp. 21–2) identifies *grant aid* alongside three other types of contract:

- *service contracts* – where there is a business-type arrangement;
- *service agreements* – where there is a closer trusting relationship and the agreement does not specify methods and inputs, but concentrates on outcomes;

- *partnership arrangements* – where there is joint provision or close co-operation between purchaser and provider.

These alternatives are valuable. The Official Guidance does not limit authorities to service contracts, and indeed encourages co-operation, to deliver a 'seamless' service. Yet Sue Lewis's account (1993), discussed above, suggests that local authorities are over-emphasising the contract as against partnership. Flynn (1993) quotes Sako's distinction of three kinds of trust: *contractual trust*, where the purchaser only trusts the provider to supply according to the contract; *competence trust*, where the purchaser buys the managerial and specialist expertise of the provider; and *goodwill trust*, where the purchaser trusts that the provider will act honourably according to the spirit of the agreement. There is a strong case for more of the latter two forms in community care policy. Common and Flynn (1992) studied how contracting was progressing in twelve authorities, showing that the degree of formality in relationships was highest at the contract-letting stage, and then tailed off into a period of rising and falling contention around control and independence. One half-way house between grant aid and a service contract is a 'service-level' agreement. This states in more detail than is customary for grant aid the amount of service to be provided (for example, hours a day centre is open, numbers of clients to be dealt with, types of problem dealt with).

Common and Flynn's (1992) study found that most contracts had started out as a result of people who knew each other and already worked together. The contracts were usually worked out jointly. The purchaser–provider split was not strongly pursued by authorities in the sample, but the fact that this policy was there had led to a greater degree of formality. Many of the contracts were to gain access to the provider's services, rather than specifying numbers of clients. A DoH study (DoH, 1993d) suggests that contracting was in the early stages still not very responsive to patterns of need emerging from assessments. Difficulties also arose for voluntary organisations in moving from grant-aided to contracting arrangements (see Chapter 9).

This survey accords with the fairly general experience of a slow start to the more marketised approach that the government has sought. Generally, existing relationships have been built up and organised on a different basis, rather than a 'contract culture' being imposed anew on the social services sector. This suggests that the social work role in its community social work/social care planning aspect will focus on helping community groups and groups of carers and users to find ways of getting into relationship with the purchasing side of agencies. Consortia and other forms of mutual support among smaller groups will also be useful.

In care management and similar roles, social workers need to take up the responsibility of feeding back to contracting staff in the local authority their experience of existing services and any knowledge of new services and operators. This makes an important contribution to keeping purchasing staff (who may easily become divorced from the field and concentrate on servicing their existing contracts rather than developing the range of possibilities for users) in touch with needs. In this way, social workers can also make a contribution to the quality assurance aspect of contracting.

Quality assurance

Two aspects of quality assurance are relevant. The concern of this part of the chapter is the general provision attached to the local authority's purchasing arrangements. The final section of the chapter deals with the other aspect, the monitoring and evaluation aspect of the care management function.

The Official Guidance (DoH/SSI, 1991) identifies three aspects of quality systems:

- *quality assurance* – in which definitions of adequate and good services are built into contracts and services and arrangements made for monitoring how standards are reached;
- *quality control* – the process of verifying that standards are met; and
- *total quality management* – a system whereby all parts of an organisation form an integrated system for constantly reviewing and enhancing the quality of their work. This is often associated with a British Standard (BS 5750) which provides for approval of organisations which have specified quality management systems; this is similarly related to an international standard (ISO 9000) (Taylor and Vigars, 1993).

Only the last is concerned with *improving* quality; the first two with specifying and maintaining it. An AMA (1991) study identifies two components of quality:

● *fitness for purpose*; and
● *standards* – which include both value and policy objectives such as choice, and social justice and practice requirements such as reliability.

Who should set standards is important, as is how they should do it and how they should assess the extent to which they have been met. Integral to this should be equality of opportunity, including taking on the particular needs of identifiable groups, particularly if they are likely to be discriminated against.

Flynn and Miller (1991) argue that providing for users and carers should be the main focus, and that therefore they should be involved in setting standards, and their needs should be the focus of professional and managerial standards. It is easy to forget in devising evaluative systems to make arrangements for maintaining accountability to the service user, by building their responses into checks on service attainments. Pfeffer and Coote (1991) argue that approaches to quality assurance imported from commercial settings are unsuitable for use in public services, although ideas like fitness for purpose, responsiveness and empowerment, borrowed from various commercial methods, can make a contribution. They argue for a 'democratic' approach in which the main purpose is equity (giving each person an equal opportunity to benefit) responding to personal needs and making the public more powerful in the definition of needs and systems. Different forms of management, which involve workers in decision-making, and provide choice to service users, participation in planning and clear rights within an open system of decision-making, are essential for this approach to quality assurance.

Despite this kind of commentary, the typical quality management relationship is a monitoring process between contracts staff in the authority and the provider. The care manager, and perhaps other local authority workers who come into contact with the provider, will gain informal impressions through their relationships, and may give advice and feedback to the contract manager. Again, because of their direct contact with service users, they are in a stronger position to maintain accountability to service users than planning and evaluation staff. Where the contract is more of a partnership, contract monitoring may be more informal (Common and Flynn, 1992, pp. 20–3).

The Official Guidance (DoH/SSI, 1991, pp. 30–6) identifies quality issues at each of four stages of contracting. When services are being specified, standards should be agreed alongside them. These may refer to inputs or outputs from the service, but might also include outcomes (not how many cases were dealt with, which would be outputs, but what was *achieved* in them), process standards (for example, speed of response, proportion of satisfied service users), and information about complaints and how they were resolved. Another feature that implies standards is the availability of mechanisms for user and carer involvement and 'customer care' policies. After standards are specified, the Guidance proposes that they should be written into the contracts, and be an essential part of the process of selection. When the contract is operating, the achievement of the agreed standards should be monitored, and action taken if they are not achieved. These can be related to complaints mechanisms (see Chapter 7).

Monitoring may involve the use of indicators, which have been controversial, because in a personal service such as social services, facts and figures can seem an inadequate way of checking standards. Warburton (1993), discussing this issue, argues that indicators can provide indications, and no more than that, of areas which might be more carefully explored. He shows that population-level comparisons have been helpful in evaluating the planning for community care, that trends in demand and service give useful indicators of need, and that practice-related indicators can be derived from inspection work, if this is systematised. Other methods of monitoring contracts are *compliance* monitoring which checks that the basic requirements are met (for example, check every so often that the day centre is open at the agreed times), *customer surveys*, *inspection* and periodic *self-evaluations* (such as annual reports) and regular *reviews* – both of clients' progress, which can be aggregated to form a view of a service, and of services provided. These again have the benefit of maintaining a focus on user accountability rather than just accountability to the commissioner of the service. Formal reviews might be done by a team of people, including care managers, members of staff and management of the provider and contract staff in the authority. Sometimes, it can be helpful to include an element of independent involvement from an outsider (for example, another authority, research from a consultant or university).

One of the problems in long-term care is making sure that standards do not slip when changes in clients' condition is relatively slow, or when maintaining care rather than therapeutic improvements is the expected form of provision. It is easy to slip into a routinised way of working which does not deal with clients' individual needs and wishes. Ammentorp *et al.* (1991) present an attractive approach to quality management in long-term care, which tries to deal with some of these difficulties. The environment within which clients receive services is conditioned, in their model, by the regulations and requirements of contracts and legislation, and also by the quality culture, meaning the attitude and group commitment of staff to maintaining quality. They distinguish between the quality of care (ie services provided) and the quality of life experienced by the client. These can and should be regularly assessed internally and by external checks. It is then important to distinguish between resolving clients' problems and resolving problems in delivering services, and to set up systems for examining each. The team working with a client concentrates on resolving personal difficulties. Separately, a quality care 'circle' – comprising people from different client care teams – meets to assess and work on service delivery problems.

Inspection and regulation

The *NHS&CCA, 1990*, made provision for changes in the regulation and inspection of residential care, which were brought into force in 1991. This was a response to a recognised problem highlighted by the Wagner Report (1988) on residential care, which had recommended changes because of inconsistency between the treatment of local authority and independent sector residential care homes. Local authorities were required to set up 'arm's-length' inspection units, separated from the management of the provision within SSDs. The units had to produce an independent annual report on their findings. According to the Policy Guidance (DoH, 1990) inspection units might develop positive roles of training and quality enhancement. A consultation document followed by a Circular (DoH, 1994b) encouraged greater openness, including publication of reports and an annual report, the appointment of lay assessors and advisory panels involving users and carers of services in reviewing inspection.

These units are important within community care policy in that they inspect and regulate a major aspect of the provision which is included in residential care. Since virtually all providers of residential care will be inspected, this forms a useful feedback and constraint on contracting with approved homes. Potentially, the inspection model could be applied to other aspects of the community care system (for example, day and domiciliary care) especially if substantial elements of these were privatised or private provision grew up. Against the extension of the inspection model is the government's wish to reduce the amount of 'red tape', particularly that affecting small businesses, which may militate against expanding regulation.

Care management monitoring

So far, in this chapter, we have been exploring district-wide service monitoring. However, we have noted several times how this relates to and affects the care management role. The fourth aspect of care management in the Official Guidance (SSI/SWSG 1991a) is monitoring; the fifth is reviewing. This distinguishes respectively between checking on and adjusting the implementation of the care plan as it affects clients, and the periodic review of the outcomes (meaning how the client has been affected, not just what has been provided) of the service package, perhaps leading to a major change in the plan. In the pre-Griffiths system, services were arranged and then very rarely adjusted unless there was a major change in circumstances. This meant that crises were often reached unnecessarily. The lack of periodic review in many adults' cases meant that they drifted with very little strategic thought about 'what next?' Monitoring and review in care management is designed to overcome both of these problems.

The monitoring and adjustment of the implementation of a care plan necessarily involves all those who participate in it. It may be inappropriate or impossible to bring all of them together on a regular basis, and so any plan needs to have communication systems built into it. The most important of these will be:

● *involvement at the planning stage* – so that everyone is aware of the starting point;
● *handover arrangements* – so that one carer can pass over

information about what has happened during the period that he
or she has been responsible;

● *support and protection arrangements* (see Chapter 5) – which
emphasise availability and responsiveness to demands;

● *confirmation of contact arrangements* – so that key stakeholders
in the care plan can get in touch with one another quickly;

● *arrangements for routine feedback* – so that people feel it is a
natural part of the process to report back on difficulties; otherwise people tend to hold back for fear of seeming critical.

Social workers often think of monitoring arrangements as requiring
home visits to question clients and carers. This may be so, but many
other possibilities are available. A quick regular telephone call to
carers and clients may be a possibility. So also may a regular letter,
or the return of a questionnaire. Clients and carers may be asked to
keep logs of any significant points, and these can be actively reviewed. Whoever is involved in the plan should be identified and a
special arrangement for monitoring their contribution can be worked
out. Timescales for monitoring are also important. In discussing the
implementation of the plan, in Chapter 6, I suggested seeing different stages of the plan's implementation as 'gates' in the pathway of
a user, when different providers join the package or a different direction is taken in the plan. These are ideal points at which to plan
monitoring.

Raiff and Shore (1993) make a number of points about good
monitoring practice. They emphasise the importance of cross-checking
different points of view. They suggest deciding on a schedule of
checks and ensuring that they are carried out. This does not rule
out responding to situations that arise, and occasionally checking
things unexpectedly. Clients and carers should be encouraged to take
part actively in the monitoring, perhaps taking on keeping a log or
handing out questionnaires themselves. They and other informal carers
could be helped to devise their own checks. Even if this is done, an
occasional review of clients' and carers' overall feelings of satisfaction is also useful. This could involve the regular administration
of questionnaires or tests of functioning for some clients, to see
how they have improved. It is important to commit time and administrative resources to monitoring, as well as to planning and
delivery of service. Administrative staff can help maintain checking
schedules and collate information, for example. Finally, Raiff and

Shore emphasise the value of monitoring all services and activities in the case, even where there is no immediate opportunity of influencing them.

The longer-term review stage of care management requires a different approach to that of monitoring. Here, the view should be strategic. What has been achieved for the client? What is the right direction now? How have views and attitudes among those involved changed? What are their wishes, especially those of clients and carers, now? Where workers are dealing with long-term care, analysis of trends, in behaviour or clients' function, may be necessary to see where progress has been made or deterioration experienced.

In the reviewing process, a formal meeting or process, involving key stakeholders in the care and clients and carers directly, gives the matter importance. It may help clients and carers to identify achievements which would otherwise have been too slight for them to notice and this may have a good effect on their motivation. Explicit plans to feed back to planners, other providers and budget-holder may be useful. Repeating some aspects of assessment and re-establishing a care plan may be useful parts of the process of review or of its outcomes.

Accountability problems

The fact that post-Griffiths community care policy contains substantial provision for monitoring and quality enhancement does not avoid other problems in accountability. We have noted how central government, although increasing the strength of its push to implement the policy effectively, loses control over the detail of implementation by fragmenting the system. Similar consequences also exist for the local authority. Although it has the responsibility for leading the planning, the requirement to involve other agencies more widely and to promote independent sector activity means that it has to manage a more complex system and a more complex planning process, and has less control over the outcome. The may be the reason for the anxiety to enforce a contract culture, noted by Sue Lewis (1993) rather than rely on trust, partnership and co-operation.

The contracting process also makes the responsibility of service providers less certain. In the pre-Griffiths system, the owner of a private old people's home knew (given the attainment of the basic standard for registration of the home) that her accountability was to the person who paid; often the client herself, sometimes a relative. In the post-Griffiths system, contracting and contract compliance, and the involvement of the care manager, user, carer, and whoever makes additional contributions to pay for the care, all have a part to play in the accountability that the owner feels. This is a more realistic range of interests, but it is harder to understand and the power of the contracting process in particular may get in the way of according most concern to the needs of clients and their carers.

We noted in Chapters 3 and 6 how the official guidance on collaboration between agencies and within the multi-disciplinary team, respectively, sought to emphasise the importance of clarity of responsibility. In reality, this is problematic. There may be a contract between the social services department and the health authority, but this cannot specify how professionals should respond to the needs of a client presented to them. The care management assessment, we saw in Chapter 4, does not guarantee that a residential care home or a nurse will agree with the overall plan, or feel accountable to a care plan produced elsewhere. The professional duties of the people involved in implementing the care plan, the wish of their organisations to retain control of their resources, and the government's demand for clarity of accountability within the services, is likely to deny accountability to the client's needs as assessed by the plan or as stated by the client. Limitations of finance and government policy to promote independence detract from the service user's right to choice within the system.

The fact that these problems of accountability exist lead inevitably to the conclusion that if the post-Griffiths system is to work effectively, co-operation and joint working will be needed at all levels of the service. One important area of quality assurance, therefore, will be the specification of co-operation and joint working within contracts, monitoring the effectiveness of joint working, and planning joint working into the system. It is to this latter aspect of community care that we turn in the final chapter.

9

Policy Development and Training for Community Care

A policy and practice innovation like community care must be prepared, go through a phase of development and early growth, and then mature. So it is not possible to describe post-Griffiths community care as complete and final. To understand practice within it, therefore, workers need to understand how the policy is developing and changing, and they need to prepare themselves for future changes. Systems of policy development and training and how they work are therefore a crucial part of practising in community care.

There are two levels of policy development to be explored: the national and the local. These are covered in the next two sections of this chapter. The third section is concerned with training. In conclusion, the final section looks at where these developments may lead community care in the future.

National policy development

Many developments in social services policy are more closely monitored and clearly pursued in the 1990s than they were in the 1970s: community care is one of them. Both the DoH and other national bodies have taken a close interest in planning for, furthering and monitoring the implementation of the policy.

DoH activity includes the following.

- *Circulars and books of guidance about implementation* – I have argued in several places in this book that such guidance, while often professionally competent and useful, directs attention and activity towards implementation of government policy, rather than necessarily conveying independent advice or covering all the possibilities.
- *Monitoring reports* – indicating progress on matters of concern to the DoH, such as the involvement of the independent sector (KPMG Management Consulting, 1992). These are often investigations over a short space of time carried out by management or academic consultants.
- *Activities by its SSI* – in giving advice and at one point organising support teams to assist local authorities whose progress in implementation was slow.
- *Research* – on aspects of the system and client groups, carers and their problems which are carried out over a longer period and are more comprehensive in their coverage of their topic. These are often undertaken from a medical or academic base. A summary of many of these are included in a compendium edited by Robbins (1993). Some of them are not concerned with community care policy as such, but refer to client groups or types of service which fall within its ambit. Many of the longer-term studies cover periods before the policy was implemented, but still provide useful information.

Each of these types of document, where they are relevant and of more than short-term interest, have been referred to in this book.

Different approaches to planning have been identified (Dean, 1991):

- *user-led* – which excludes non-users, whose needs may also be significant and different from those of known users;
- *needs-led* – which creates difficulties in defining and measuring needs at a general level; and
- *outcome-led* – which also produces difficulties in definition and measurement, and fails to focus on how services will go about meeting needs, since good-quality services are likely to be concerned about methods and process as much as outcome.

Other national bodies have taken an interest in various aspects of community care. These include the following.

- *Research and development organisations* An example is the Kings Fund, which has a concern for health service issues, and has undertaken research and published surveys of literature. It has also tackled projects of particular relevance to community care, although they started with a more general base; an example is the 'informal caring programme' (Richardson *et al.* 1989; Robinson and Yee, 1991). Other examples of such organisations are the Joseph Rowntree Foundation, which has funded a research programme and series of publications on 'Community Care into Practice' (for example, Common and Flynn, 1992); and the National Institute for Social Work, some of whose longer-term research work on elders has been relevant, and which has also provided consultancy services from time to time. Another active group has been the Nuffield Institute for Health Service Studies in Leeds (for example, Wistow *et al.*, 1993).
- *Specialist community care groups* These include those with a particular concern for issues relevant to community care. The national (and to some extent local) private residential care homes organisations have been active in pressing the need for their interests to be taken into account.
- *General lobbying and professional bodies* These have pursued their particular interests. The British Association of Social Workers has, as a relatively small part of its activities, issued some policy materials on community care designed to press the role of social workers as part of the policy (BASW, nd). Others have taken up particular aspects relevant to their expertise. The Child Poverty Action Group, for example, has published welfare rights guidance on various problems which have arisen in helping people with the social security consequences of receiving community care services (Thompson, P., 1992; CRO, 1993). Many organisations with connections in the social services and health worlds have represented points of view or interests.

All these groups form a network of national interactions concerned to push forward community care policy, and add something of their own slant to it. There are also different national perspectives. Hunter and Wistow (1987) show how different national histories and differing policies in the Scottish and Welsh Offices led to markedly different policy moves in the 1980s. Bodies such as the Welsh Health Planning Forum, established within the NHS (Riley, 1993) suggests that varying structures will always have differing effects throughout the UK. An important distinction in Northern Ireland has always been the fact that social services are part of the health services structure (and therefore open for trust status) rather than being a local authority service. This should, but does not always, permit better relationships with health provision, while placing obstructions in relationships with local authorities. Links and obstructions always need to be carefully explored, and ways of responding to them worked out by practitioners.

Within the interest networks, social work organisations are not predominant. The most influential of these is probably the SSI which, although it is aware of social work issues, obviously presses government policy rather than an independent professional line. At the outset, much of the influence has gone to those concerned with setting up the management and contracting systems, such as representatives of employers' organisations and management consultants and researchers. This is not surprising, in view of the initial need to set up arrangements for making local community care plans, rather than implementing the practice elements of community care. Concern for practice within the system has been limited, it being assumed that care management is a managerial and procedural activity, and that social work practice, in so far as it is relevant, would continue as before.

The future development of social work practice with client groups and using the skills particularly relevant to community care will, however, require a stronger concern for the development of effective practice options, if service users are not to be left in the community without adequate support. We have seen in previous chapters how careful and creative application of a range of social work therapeutic/counselling and community social work/social care planning roles and skills is needed to fulfil the potential of community care policy. It is crucial that government and agencies have serious plans for stimulating and developing practice policy to permit this.

In addition to standard services, the government has made 'specific grants' to develop particular aspects of community care services which are considered to be underdeveloped. Provisions for two types of grant for mental illness and drugs and alcohol services were inserted into Section 7 of the *Local Authority Social Services Act, 1970* by Section 50 of the *NHS&CCA, 1990* (DoH, 1990, pp. 19–20). A report (SSI, 1993) on the implementation of the mental illness specific grant argues that, while resources have been small, it has encouraged joint work among agencies and allowed a number of useful services to be developed for an appreciable number of users. From time to time, other special projects are devised. One example is the 'Caring for People who Live at Home' initiative announced in 1992, which seeks to encourage new domiciliary and day services in the independent sector, where, particular among private providers, residential provision has in the past been the main focus (Allen, 1993; DoH, 1992b). Such schemes, again, focus effort on meeting the government's objectives to promote its management approach of competition and diversity.

Local policy development

Local policy development also takes place within a network of interests, but is focused around the annual preparation of the community care plan for the area. This is usually undertaken by the SSD in close liaison with the health authority and should involve other relevant authorities and agencies as well. Wistow *et al.*'s study (1993) of a sample of early plans showed that most were prepared by some joint process, a few more were jointly approved and many others were broadly complementary. Only a few seemed to have been prepared entirely within the SSD. In a later study of the 1993/4 plans (Hardy *et al.*, 1993, p. 4) better consultation was in evidence, and a few authorities had 'highly developed inter-agency relationships'. Arrangements were said to be working better than in the previous history of joint planning. Where plans are not prepared jointly, agencies should have 'planning agreements' as the basis of co-operation (DoH, 1990, pp. 14–15). DoH advice is that jointness should not affect the clarity of the accountability of social services and health authorities for their provision (DoH, 1990, p. 15). Planning should also involve the 'independent sector', both voluntary organisations, which have generally been fairly well represented, and private organisations, whose participation has been patchy (KPMG Management Consulting, 1992). As a result, the Secretary of State issued directions in 1993 requiring local authorities to consult representative organisations that notified the local authority of their wish to be involved (DoH, 1993a), another indication of the concern to make the marketised management approach of the government work. As well as this, the ideals of post-Griffiths policy require the involvement of users and carers organisations. Sometimes these are participants because their organisations seek to provide services as well as represent users' and carers' interests. Some voluntary sector organisations would also claim to represent users' and carers' interests, but it is sometimes unclear whether they have representative systems or advocacy schemes which allow them to represent users' and carers' views (which might well be different from what the organisation conceives of as their interests).

Planning processes of this type seem very distant from the everyday role of social workers, whether they are care managers or service providers, and there is evidence, for example in services for young people with disabilities, that conceptions of the overall service do not filter down from senior to middle management and on to fieldwork staff (DoH, 1993f). However, they may be able to contribute their experience of needs and services and the way they work in practice to working parties. It may be important to establish that a practitioner input to such planning processes can reflect realities in a way that looking at statistics and representing interests does not. One study (SSI/NHSME, 1993) suggested that, at least in the early stages, local authorities were not aggregating information about users' decisions to help them decide on future developments. One 'community social work/social care planning' role of social workers may be to assist organisations of users and carers to set themselves up and help to ensure that they become part of the planning system.

One important aspect of local policy implementation is co-operation between local authorities and health authorities on discharge from hospital, since an early fear was that local authorities would not have an incentive to help health authorities reduce pressure on beds and there might be disputes about local authorities paying for nursing homes. Local agreements (called 'December 1992' agreements following on from a DoH circular – DoH, 1992d) were supposed to cover detailed arrangements about this, and for the relationship between hospital and community social workers; they have proved generally effective in avoiding problems (DoH, 1993c).

Health services should not be the only agencies involved, although the government guidance, produced by the DoH, tends to give priority to them. Discharge from hospitals, particularly of long-stay patients, and community care generally requires also careful attention to housing provision and a shared agenda there (Fletcher, 1993).

Jamieson (1991), comparing Danish and British community care provision for older people, comments that British problems with housing for this client group are just as severe as in Denmark, but government policy does not want to give a prominent role for housing within state provision. Pinch (1993) argues that there should also be attempts to overcome barriers to receiving care among homeless people. A government circular (DoE/DoH, 1992) emphasises the importance of housing provision and promotes joint involvement in planning and assessment. Housing strategies should take community care needs into account.

According to the official guidance (DoH, 1990, pp. 11–20), plans should include statements of objectives and targets, but only within national policy (p. 17); arrangements for assessment; the services they intend to provide and priorities among them; how they are going to ensure quality and consumer choice; and information about resources, including improving cost-effectiveness, consultation and how information is to be published. The emphasis on priorities, quality, consumers and cost-effectiveness all reflect the government's management approach to public services in general and show how it is being implemented within community care. The plans are supposed to be supported by 'hard data' presented in an accessible way (p. 20). Among the contributors to such data would be a 'population needs assessment' by which the planners would identify what needs were likely to be relevant to the population in their area. Official guidance for undertaking these assessments (Price Waterhouse, 1993) advises that statistical information applying to the general population and information about the local area from a variety of agencies should be combined to show what groups of people are likely to be in the area and what problems they are likely to suffer from. This helps to indicate what quantity and type of services will be required. Workers can usefully make sure that planners know if they have any population data which may not be known to the department. A local organisation may have carried out a small survey, for example.

Following planning, local authorities have to implement their policies. This requires them to develop a continuing relationship with providers in their areas. Difficulties here include the fact that independent sector provision is not well-developed in many areas, and that there is a conflict between a need to give all care providers a chance to offer services, while protecting those – particularly voluntary organisations – which might be adversely affected by market pressures, and the need to support new services in the early stages, while maintaining cost-effective services and not implying favouritism to particular services (DoH, 1993d). The process of making, maintaining and monitoring contracts, discussed in Chapter 8, is an integral part of implementing planning.

An important aspect of the planning process now that community care has been implemented is that feedback from the system should contribute to future plans. A good planning system will therefore have arrangements to identify demands on the service, and particularly needs which are assessed but not met, or which are not met in the ideal way. Wide availability of information about costs will enhance decision-making at the planning level and where workers are making decisions about appropriate provision (Netten and Beecham, 1993; Beecham and Netten, 1993). An important role of care managers is to find ways of feeding information of this kind back to planners, and if there is no system for this, making sure information is passed on and agitating for a system to be set up. Social workers who are providing care management or helping services may also consider encouraging users and carers to offer similar feedback. This might be a useful focus for stimulating organisations of users and carers.

A further 'community social work/social care planning' role of a social worker may be to participate in creating a new voluntary or private organisation to offer a service or an approach which is missing and would be valued. Many voluntary sector organisations have developed through the specialist interests and commitment of social workers, and the effort to create wider community care services as post-Griffiths policy is implemented offers some flexible opportunities to get these financed. Some of the skills referred to in Chapters 6 and 7 can be helpful here. In particular, alliances across organisational and professional divides can help to stimulate new ideas and activities.

Training

Training structures and policy

As post-Griffiths community care policy was an attempt at innovation in social work practice and social services policy, it was evi-

Figure 9.1 *Training structures and policies*

Initial training	Agency training	Post-qualifying training
for new workers	*for experienced workers*	*for experienced workers*
Basic practice skills		Advanced practice skills
Understanding of multi-disciplinary work	Experience of multi-disciplinary work with joint training	Multi-disciplinary joint training
Community care practice skills	Community care practice skills	Community care practice skills

dent from an early stage that additional training would be required. Various developments and policies fit together in a structure set out in Figure 9.1; some of the structure is, as we shall see, already in place – more of it is potential or planned.

Official guidance looks mainly at training within agencies. In one DoH circular, among the key tasks identified for completion in the financial year 1992/3 was 'ensuring that staff are suitably trained, wherever appropriate on a joint basis' (DoH, 1992c, Annex B). Guidance was issued on organising joint training (DoH, 1991), and the Audit Commission (1992b, p. 35), in reviewing how the changes were being implemented in the early stages, emphasised how important training in new skills would be, in addition to keeping staff well-informed. Joint training, in particular, could help to forge new links between services, overcoming traditional differences and conflicts between professional groups (Weinstein, 1994). Additional grant aid for training was provided for SSDs.

Further guidance was issued in 1993 (DoH, 1993b) which was less concerned to promote methods of joint training, but more to present training for the implementation of community care as a process in stages. This emphasises the importance of managing training effectively, planning for it over the long term and assessing and strengthening the capability of the agencies involved to provide effective training. Concern is expressed (p. 37) about the high turnover of management and training staff, which reduces training capability. Bell (1993) similarly emphasises that training is an important resource which needs careful planning. In particular she argues (p. 25) that plans for developing the organisation need to go hand-in-hand with plans for staff and management development, and that defining organisational needs should be congruent with staff definitions of their own needs. She proposes a complex consultation process aligning staff's definitions of their needs with managerial definitions of the organisation's needs before a training plan can be worked out.

The official guidance and associated commentary is concerned mainly with training of existing staff as part of the development and implementation of policy within agencies. Much agency training is likely to be focused on operational needs – what the agency requires in order to carry out its policies and objectives. Of equal concern is the provision of training

- incorporating current community care practice into initial training for social workers;
- offering more extensive advanced training, possibly along with qualifications, to qualified workers either in
  — community care practice, management and policy; or
  — specialised practice relating to client groups covered by community care policy.

This latter distinction is important. Courses providing for training in, say, care management and budgeting may be useful for people fulfilling those roles, and may well be an early priority in order to help get the policy running effectively. However, in the longer term, in the same way that I have argued that practice policy needs to develop, practice training also needs to develop so that workers have sophisticated options to provide creative and stimulating choices for their clients in the community. A long-term study (Mansell and Beasley, 1993) of small houses for people with learning difficulties and challenging behaviour showed, for example, that good standards of provision and considerable progress for clients could be achieved, but this was difficult to maintain without constant development of staff skill and commitment. Similarly, if residential care is to have a future as a non-stigmatised choice for service users, creative forms of involvement and stimulation for residents will be required. The impact of treatment innovations will be much enhanced by more widespread opportunities for training focused on the needs of particular groups of people in need, as well as management and care structures. Another advantage of focusing on particular client groups is the opportunity for training multi-disciplinary groups of workers together around the interests and needs of the group of people for whom they jointly provide.

Although for clarity in Figure 9.1, I have presented both initial and post-qualifying training separately from agency training, current systems of education organised by CCETSW stress the importance of partnership between specialised training providers, so that agencies are likely to be co-operating with and can influence the content and methods of initial training, even where this is based in universities and colleges. Agencies in many areas also participate in joint post-qualifying schemes and can contribute modules to wider qualifications drawing on their own specialist expertise and experience.

Another important part of training structures in community care is the opportunity afforded by joint training, whether within agencies for operational purposes or within post-qualifying structures for wider developmental purposes, for joint training between different sectors, as well as between different specialist disciplines. Voluntary and private sector agencies often do not have the resources or numbers of staff with shared needs to be able to mount training on their own behalf, and the possibility exists of including them within social service or health authority training provision. This might make such courses broader in perspective and be an effective way of making links between the sectors. Similarly, initial training, which currently focuses on local authority experience as a common denominator, may need to include more material on the different sectors and links between them.

Content and methods: knowledge, skills and values

The training structures and policies set out in Figure 9.1 suggest that different kinds of content are required in community care training:

• practice skills with particular client groups, aspects of need and methods of practice;

- multi-disciplinary work; and
- community care policies and practice, which will include:
  — a significant element of management, and
  — professional care management skills, which include many elements of practice skills concerned with assessment, planning and implementing and monitoring care plans, which I have argued require development of social work skills.

Knowledge about client groups or others involved, such as carers, and possible methods of work to meet their needs, appears first in this list because in generic SSD's specialised knowledge about long-term care needs has not been strongly valued. Before the Griffiths community care reforms, assessment required only a fairly cursory understanding of needs in order to fit them with the limited range of services available. More detailed understanding of various disabilities, the consequences of learning difficuilties or experiences of later life are required to understand the full implications of an infinitely variable package of services. More thoughtful understanding of the implications of the situations of clients is required to negotiate over a range of possibilities rather than specify a set service. Various examples and research quoted throughout this book have indicated that good knowledge of clients' problems and of services is valued by clients and necessary for effective work. The implication of this is, eventually, an emphasis on specialised learning for many occupations in SSDs which have relied on generic knowledge rather than a detailed appreciation of personal and service needs for particular client groups.

Service provision within the package which is offered also requires greater understanding of clients' limitations and opportunities together with the variety of methods which might be available to meet them. This is particularly important where clients are mainly in their own homes, because where they are in day or residential care there is a variety of workers with different skills available to offer various treatment options. Also, the environment is more stimulating, because there are more people, more and more variety of options for movement and placing yourself, and clients have moved to it from their own homes so it offers 'difference'. Clients receiving domiciliary services can find themselves staring at the wall in their own homes with very little variation in experience or people coming to see them: this requires much more stimulation and a wider range of opportunities.

Every area should, therefore, have opportunities for building knowledge about different client groups covered by community care, and for building knowledge and understanding of the needs of carers, volunteers and other personnel likely to be involved. There should also be methodology training which offers opportunities to draw on ideas like reminiscence therapy, music, art and occupational therapies to provide stimulation and development for clients. It is also important to develop workers' skills in community social work activities, such as stimulating user and carer groups and promoting volunteer and informal care groups in the community. If post-Griffiths community care policy is to be effective, this community level of work is just as crucial as skills in care management and with individual clients.

Multi-disciplinary work is often seen as the basis for all forms of co-operation between workers and agencies in community care. However, we saw in Chapter 6 that official policy on collaboration was concerned with identifying accountability and that this led to a view of collaboration which focused on defining boundaries between occupational groups involved in community care. Much research on multi-disciplinary work seems to show that a clear understanding of agreed boundaries but a preparedness to blur roles across those boundaries is essential to effective joint working. Training in this area, therefore, needs to focus on both clarity and jointness. There is a danger that proposing joint training as the basis for community care working on the assumption that it must be multi-disciplinary may lead to training being done on defining differences, without working on sharing, or working on co-operation without understanding boundaries properly.

In Chapter 6, we also noted that joint working required skills in linking and liaison which were demanded among different elements of services and between agencies or parts of them. Multi-disciplinary training, joint or otherwise, will not therefore furnish all the skills required for effective community care work.

That management skills are an integral part of effective community care work may seem obvious, in view of all the discussion about budgeting, delegation of responsibility, planning and liaison work. However, I think it is important to distinguish aspects of work concerned with the management of the service undertaken by various people involved in community care provision from the professional skills involved in *care* management. For example, financial assessment, feedback to community care plans, managing groups of staff and informal carers making provision for clients, are all crucial elements of provision and require organisational and personnel management skills which go beyond self-management and care planning and implementation. Management training which focuses on managing groups of people, financial skills and communication skills is important: personal skills such as time and stress management may also be useful.

The central chapters of this book have focused on community care skills such as assessment, care planning, plan implementation, monitoring and advocacy for clients. These particular skills associated with post-Griffiths community care need to be developed, and their content better understood and made a more integral part of social work practice in community care. It is a corollary of the argument of this book that skills of linking, liaison, assessment, planning, monitoring and advocacy can and should be taught explicitly, rather than being taken for granted as something that most competent adults possess or which are common sense. Post-Griffiths community care policy requires a high level of skill in integrating clients with services. This is partly because of the ideal of choice and of a tailored care package. It also arises because the government's chosen management style, promoting competition and marketisation, seems likely to create a fragmented and confusing range of services, even though it might have the potential to create greater variety and opportunity. Care managers will, therefore, have to exhibit skills of a high order if clients are to take advantage of the possibilities while not being disadvantaged by the consequences of this management policy.

The future for community care

In Chapter 2, I identified three historical aims of community care. If, in concluding this book, I am to make any judgements about the possibilities for community care, I need to distinguish between them.

The original aim of community care was to remove mentally ill people and people with learning disabilities from long-term institutional care wherever possible and provide alternatives for them in the community. This element of the policy has been progressing for decades and in many ways can be regarded as almost complete.

The achievements are that most people who were in long-term care who could be discharged have been or soon will be, and many of them are happier, and are not too much of a burden on their families and their informal carers or the community around them (see, for example, Simic, 1994, Petch, 1994). Most people whose mental illness is active do not receive institutional care to the point where they become dependent on it, although there are a few who become long-stay patients. Because their illness is active, they present more difficulties to relatives and carers, and a number are not regularly in contact with psychiatric services or receiving appropriate support. On a few occasions, they end up on the street and in the prisons. Short-stay hospitals do not want to provide for them, because there is little to be done about their care needs, and they want to avoid long-term institutionalisation.

Efforts are being made by government to develop clear structures for the supervision of this group. Proposals include a supervised discharge arrangement for patients who do not take medication or comply with a treatment programme, and a register of patients at risk. This latter idea responds in part to the Christopher Clunis Enquiry into a case where man with a history of mental disorder committed a murder, in spite of the fact that he was known to many agencies, but with none co-ordinating a response (Ritchie, 1994). Considerable resources and some re-orientation of the conventional approach of short-stay psychiatric treatment to organise better co-ordination will be needed to make it effective. The Mansell Committee (1993), which gives advice on dealing with people with mental health problems and learning disabilities who also present challenging behaviour, argues that there is enough experience available to identify the main principles of providing a safe, effective service for people with relatively severe difficulties. They identify three types of service objective: *removal*, which seeks to remove people with such difficulties from local services; *containment*, where they are accepted, but only contained within low cost, poor-quality services; and *development*, where the aim is to address individual needs. Important features of such services are that they individualise people presenting severe behaviour difficulties to services, rather than labelling them as difficult; define their role in relation to such people clearly; find an effective middle ground between pessimism and optimism; and concentrate on good relationships and networking, so that challenging behaviour is not worsened by discontinuity in service and poor communication.

The future for this aim of community care is to wait for the remaining elderly population of long-stay hospitals to die, helping those who are capable of independence to discharge or at least a more independent life in smaller hospital units, to provide effective 'asylum' for people with active mental illness or severe learning difficulties who need residential or hospital help, and to provide effective supervision and protection for such people whose life is mainly outside institutions and support for their carers. As the long-stay hospitals die, more resources might be released for these future needs. It remains to be seen whether those resources will continue to be dedicated to these care needs, or whether they will be seen as a useful saving to the public purse. The concerned social worker should fight for the former.

The second aim, particularly of post-Griffiths community care policy, was to resolve the 'perverse incentives' of the pre-existing social security regime for people in private residential care, which had led to the development of extensive and expensive private-sector provision in the 1980s. At the same time, the government's management approach took advantage of those private sector developments to create a 'mixed economy of care' by welding a role for the independent sector into the 'purchaser–provider split' and facilitated co-ordination at the planning level, by giving local authorities a lead role in community care planning, and developing the idea of care management.

The achievements in this area are organisationally complete, and the initial rounds of community care planning have led to fairly basic collections of existing services in the first instance, but joint planning is improving and may lead to more involving and co-ordinated plans if the pressure to maintain effective and involving planning is kept up. Although the organisation of this aspect of community care is complete, however, it is still unclear whether a wider range of services in a mixed economy will be created, or whether this will lead to improvements which will overcome the fragmentation of the previously co-ordinated local authority care system. It is also unclear whether care management has been established in such a way that the opportunities for flexibility, choice and user involvement will be achieved, rather than a bureaucratisation of the pattern of services in an unhelpful way.

To make this aspect of community care work for clients, workers will need to develop the skills to make care management an effective and responsive opportunity for clients to achieve the care package that they want. They will also need to use the skills of community social work to help create the user, carer and informal organisations' involvement in the community care planning process which will allow the system of services available to their clients to be available and appropriate to the wishes and needs of the population of the area. Managers will need to prevent the system becoming rigid and unhelpful in its organisation.

The third aim of community care is more diffuse. It is to achieve that ideal of service for people who need long-term care that makes the services they receive contribute to their independence, to the chance to lead a style and quality of life which we would all value, and to have control over the choice of how they live (especially to avoid unnecessary residential care if they want to avoid it), how they are cared for and who their carers and social contacts are.

Very little progress has been made with this aim. The range and flexibility of care services has been and is poor. The openness of public services to change, respect and opportunity for users' choice and involvement has been limited. Dependence, stigma and lack of control is a feature of the lives of many receiving caring services. Lack of support and help is the lot of many informal carers. The ideals behind the Griffiths community care reforms seek to enforce users' and carers' involvement, opportunities for choice, avoidance of unnecessary residential care and a chance for greater independence. One opportunity which has been met by the manner of reform is that provision has been left at a local level where workers, users and carers can come to know the system pretty well. The service remains within local government, so there are local political channels for lobbying if improvements need to be made; this can be a beneficial addition to or context for good management which the reforms try to stimulate.

Misgivings arise about many of these apparent opportunities. One of the objectives of the reforms is to contain expenditure. The ideal of independence may become a demand if necessary dependence incurs too much cost. The centralisation of expenditure through SSDs may remove perverse incentives, but it also discloses the full scale of caring expenditure and exposes it to cost-cutting concerns and removes choice in sources of income and support. Openness, choice, and flexibility are always limited in government guidance by cost considerations. The government's management approach may fragment and confuse services or lead to wasted resources because of competition or poor information. Provision for consumer choice and involvement, multi-disciplinary joint management and planning and the offer of care management may well overcome some of the co-ordinative lacunae of pre-existing services, but they must also surmount the steeper – perhaps the unnecessarily steep – hills of the more confused and fragmented care system which seems likely to take its place.

Much depends – as it always does – on how it is implemented on the ground. In focusing on the skills and opportunities for good practice within the community care system, I have argued in this book for the value of effective social work as part of post-Griffiths community care, and tried to show how it might be made more effective by analysis of skills and understanding of the system within which those skills must be practised. In spite of the features of the post-Griffiths system which seem likely to detract from the ideals which it seeks to achieve, hopes for future benefit for users and their carers will rely on the commitment, drive and skills with which multi-disciplinary teams can make the best use of social work in community care.

Bibliography

Abrams, Philip, Sheila Abrams, Robin Humphrey and Ray Snaith (1989) *Neighbourhood Care and Social Policy* (London, HMSO).

Ad Hoc Committee on Advocacy (1969) 'The social worker as advocate: champions of social victims', *Social Work* (14)2, pp. 16–21.

Adams, Robert (1990) *Self-help, Social Work and Empowerment* (London, Macmillan).

ADSS/SSI (1991) *Care in the Community Project: Care Management and Assessment* (London, ADSS/SSI, CITC 5).

Allan, Graham A. (1983) 'Informal networks of care: issues raised by Barclay', *British Journal of Social Work*, 13(4), pp. 417–33.

Allen, Isobel (1993) 'Introduction', in Diana Leat, *The Development of Community Care by the Independent Sector* (London, Policy Studies Institute).

Allen-Meares, Paula and B.A. Lane (1987) 'Grounding social work practice in theory: ecosystems', *Social Casework*, 68(11), pp. 517–21.

AMA (1991) *Quality and Contracts in the Personal Social Services* (London, Association of Metropolitan Authorities).

Ammentorp, William, Kenneth D. Gossett and Nancy Euchner Poe (1991) *Quality Assurance for Long-term Care Providers* (Newbury Park, CA, Sage).

Arber, Sara and Nigel Gilbert (1989) 'Men: the forgotten carers', *Sociology*, 23(1), pp. 111–18.

Askham, J. and C. Thompson (1990) *Dementia and Home Care: A research report on a home support scheme for dementia sufferers* (Survey of Age Concern, England).

Atkin, Karl (1991) 'Community care in a multi-racial society: incorporating the user view', *Policy and Politics*, 19(3), pp. 159–66.

Atkin, Karl and Janet Rollings (1993) *Community Care in a Multi-Racial Britain: a critical review of the literature* (London, HMSO).

Audit Commission (1986) *Making and Reality of Community Care* (London, HMSO).

Audit Commission (1992a) *The Community Revolution: personal social services and community care* (London, HMSO).

Audit Commission (1992b) *Community Care: Managing the Cascade of Change* (London, HMSO).

Bailey, Roy and Mike Brake (eds.) (1975) *Radical Social Work* (London, Edward Arnold).

Baldwin, Norma, John Harris and Des Kelly (1993) 'Institutionalisation: why blame the institution?', *Ageing and Society*, 13, pp. 69–81.

Baldwin, Steve (1993) *The Myth of Community Care: an alternative neighbourhood model of care* (London, Chapman & Hall).

Barclay Report (1982) *Social Workers: their role and tasks* (London, Bedford Square Press).

Barham, Peter (1992) *Closing the Asylum: the mental patient in modern society* (Harmondsworth, Penguin).

Barr, Alan (1989) 'New dog – new tricks? Some principles and implications for community social work', in Gerald Smale and William Bennett (eds), *Pictures of Practice: vol. 1 Community Social Work in Scotland* (London, National Institute for Social Work).

Bartlett, Harriet M. (1970) *The Common Base of Social Work Practice* (New York, National Association of Social Workers).

Barton, W. Russell (1959) *Institutional Neurosis* (Bristol, John Wright).

BASW (1980) *Clients are Fellow Citizens* (Birmingham, British Association of Social Workers).

BASW (nd – 1992?) *Community Care – Whose Choice?* (Birmingham, British Association of Social Workers).

Bayley, Michael J. (1973) *Mental Handicap and Community Care: a study of mentally handicapped people in Sheffield* (London, Routledge & Kegan Paul).

Bayley, Michael, J. Paul Parker, Rosalind Seyd and Alan Tennant (1987) *Practising Community Care: developing locally-based practice* (Sheffield, Social Services Monographs: Research in Practice).

Bayliss, Elizabeth (1987) *Housing: the foundation of community care* (London, National Federation of Housing Associations).

Bean, Philip and Mounser, Patricia (1993) *Discharged from Mental Hospitals* (London, Macmillan).

Beardshaw, Virginia and David Towell (1990) *Assessment and Case Management: Implications for the Implementation of 'Caring for People'* (London, King's Fund Institute, Briefing Paper 10).

Beecham Jennifer and Ann Netten (eds) (1993) *Community Care in Action: the role of costs* (Canterbury, PSSRU).

Belbin, R. Meredith (1981) *Management Teams: why they succeed or fail* (Oxford, Heinemann).

Bell, Lesley (1993) 'Developing tomorrow's managers today', *Community Care Management and Planning*, 1(1), pp. 24–8.

Beresford, Peter and Suzy Croft (1986) *Whose Welfare? private care or public services* (Brighton, Sussex, Lewis Cohen Centre for Urban Studies).

Beresford, Peter and Suzy Croft (1993) *Citizen Involvement: a practical guide for change* (London, Macmillan).

Biehal, Nina (1993) 'Changing practice: participation, rights and community care', *British Journal of Social Work*, 23(5), pp. 443–58.

Biestek, Felix P. (1965) *The Casework Relationship* (London, Allen & Unwin).

Biggs, Simon (1991) 'Community Care, case management and the psychodynamic perspective', *Journal of Social Work Practice,* 5(1), pp. 71–81.

Bland, Rosemary (1994) 'EPIC – a Scottish case management experiment', in Mike Titterton (ed.), *Caring for People in the Community: the new welfare* (London, Jessica Kingsley), pp. 113–29.

Bloor, Michael, Neil McKeganey and Dick Fonkert (1988) *One Foot in Eden: a sociological study of the range of therapeutic community practice* (London, Routledge).

Bottomley, Virginia (1990) 'Foreword', in DoH, *Community Care in the Next Decade and Beyond: Policy Guidance* (London, HMSO).

Bradshaw, Jonathan (1972) 'The taxonomy of social need', in G. McLachlan (ed.), *Problems and Progress in Medical Care* (Oxford, Oxford University Press).

Brandon, David (1989) 'The courage to look at the moon', *Social Work Today,* 50(50), pp. 16–17.

Braithwaite, Valerie A. (1990) *Bound to Care* (Sydney, Allen & Unwin).

Brearley, C. P. (1982) *Risk and Social Work* (London, Routledge & Kegan Paul).

Brenton, Maria (1985) *The Voluntary Sector in British Social Services* (London, Longman).

Brigden, Patricia and Margaret Todd (eds) (1993) *Concepts in Community Care for People with a Learning Difficulty* (London, Macmillan).

Broady, Maurice and Rodney Hedley (1989) *Working Partnerships: community development in local authorities* (London, Bedford Square Press).

Brooke, Rodney (1989) *Managing the Enabling Authority* (London, Longman).

Brown, Christopher and Charles Ringma (1989) 'New disability services: the critical role of staff in a consumer-directed empowerment model', *Disability, Handicap and Society,* 4(3), pp. 251–4.

Brown, Hilary and Helen Smith (eds) (1992) *Normalisation: a reader for the nineties* (London, Routledge).

Brown, Phil (1985) *The Transfer of Care: psychiatric deinstitutionalisation and its aftermath* (London, Routledge).

Brown, Stephen and Gerald Wistow (eds) (1990) *The Role and Tasks of Community Mental Handicap Teams* (Aldershot, Hants, Gower).

Bull, David (1982) *Welfare Advocacy: whose means to what ends?* (Birmingham, BASW Publications).

Bulmer, Martin (1986) *Neighbours: the work of Philip Abrams* (Cambridge, Cambridge University Press).

Bulmer, Martin (1987) *The Social Basis of Community Care* (London, Allen & Unwin).

Bytheway, Bill (1989) 'Poverty, care and age: a case study', in Bill Bytheway, Theresa Keil, Patricia Allatt and Alan Bryman (eds), *Becoming and Being Old: sociological approaches to later life* (London, Sage).

Cambridge, Paul and Martin Knapp (eds) (1988) *Demonstrating Successful Care in the Community* (Canterbury, Kent Personal Social Service Research Unit).

Challis, David (1994) 'Case management: a review of UK developments and issues', in Mike Titterton (ed.), *Caring for People in the Community: the new welfare* (London, Jessica Kingsley) pp. 91–112.

Challis, D., R. Chessum, J. Chesterman, R. Luckett and K. Traske (1990) *Case Management in Social and Health Care* (Canterbury, Kent, Personal Social Services Research Unit).

Challis, D., R. Chessum, J. Chesterman, R. Luckett and B. Woods (1988) 'Community care for the frail elderly: an urban experiment', in B. Davies and M. Knapp (eds), *The Production of Welfare Approach: evidence and argument from the PSSRU* Supplement to the *British Journal of Social Work*, 18, pp. 13–42.

Challis, D., R. Darton, L. Johnson, M. Stone, K. Traske and B. Wall (1989) *The Darlington Community Care Project: supporting frail elderly people at home* (Canterbury, Kent, Personal Social Services Research Unit).

Cheetham, Juliet (1993) 'The effectiveness of homemakers in housing and social work project, Castlemilk, Glasgow', in Social Work Research Centre, Stirling, *Is Social Work Effective? Research findings from the Social Work Research Centre* (Stirling, Social Work Research Centre).

Children Act, 1989.

CIPFA Competition Joint Committee (1989) *The Extension of Compulsory Competition: Meeting the Challenge: VI: Code of Practice for Compulsory Competition 1989* (London, CIPFA).

Clark, David H. (1964) *Administrative Therapy: the role of the doctor in the therapeutic community* (London, Tavistock).

Clayton, Susan (1983) 'Social need revisited' *Journal of Social Policy*, 12(2), pp. 215–34.

Cliffe, David, with David Berridge (1991) *Closing Children's Homes: an end to residential childcare?* (London, National Children's Bureau).

Cohen, Jeffrey and Mike Fisher (1988) 'Mental health and the relatives of social work clients', *Practice*, 2(2), pp. 101–19.

Collins, Alice H. and Diane L. Pancoast (1976) *Natural Helping Networks: a strategy for prevention* (Washington, DC, National Association of Social Workers).

Common, Richard and Flynn, Norman (1992) *Contracting for Care* (York, Joseph Rowntree Foundation).

Compton, Beulah Roberts (1989) 'An attempt to examine the use of support in social work practice', in Beulah R. Compton and Burt Galaway *Social Work Processes* (4th edn) (Belmont, CA, Wadsworth) pp. 564–72.

Connor, Anne (1994) 'The role of the voluntary sector in the new community care arrangements', in Mike Titterton (ed.), *Caring for People in the Community: the new welfare* (London, Jessica Kingsley) pp. 130–52.

Crow, Graham and Graham Allan (1994) *Community Life: an introduction to local social relations* (London, Harvester Wheatsheaf).

CRAG (1992, 1993, 1994) *Charging for Residential Accommodation Guide* (London, Department of Health; Cardiff, Welsh Office).

CRO (1993) 'How is community care working?', *Welfare Rights Bulletin*, 116 (October 1993), pp. 2–4.

Cumberlege Report (1986), *Neighbourhood Nursing – a focus for care* (Report of the Community Nursing Review) (London, HMSO).

Dalley, Gillian (1988) *Ideologies of Caring* (London, Macmillan).

Dalley, Gillian (1989) 'Professional ideology or organisational tribalism? the health service–social work divide', in Jan Walmsley, Jill Reynolds, Pam Shakespeare and Ray Woolfe (eds) *Health Welfare and Practice: reflecting on roles and relationships* (London, Sage).

Dalrymple, Jane (1993) Personal Communication from the Director of Advice, Advocacy and Representation Service for Children.

Darvill, Giles and Gerald Smale (eds) (1990) *Partners in Empowerment: networks of innovation in social work* (London, National Institute for Social Work).

Davis Smith, Justin (1992), 'What we know about volunteering: information from the surveys', in Rodney Hedley and Justin Davis Smith, *Volunteering and Society: principles and practice* (London, Bedford Square Press).

Davies, Bleddyn and David Challis (1986) *Matching Resources to Needs in Community Care: an evaluated demonstration of a long-term care model* (Aldershot, Hants, Gower).

Davies, Bleddyn and Martin Knapp (1988) 'Introduction: the production of welfare approach: some new PSSRU argument and results', in B. Davies and M. Knapp (eds), *The Production of Welfare Approach: evidence and argument from the PSSRU* Supplement to the *British Journal of Social Work*, 18, pp. 1–11.

Day, Peter, R. (ed.) (1993) *Perspectives on Later Life* (London, Whiting & Birch).

Dean, Malcolm (1991) 'Seamless service or fragile market?' *Search*, 8, pp. 4–6.

DHSS (1976) *Joint Care Planning: health and local authorites* (London, DHSS Circular [HC(76)18, LAC(76)6]).

DHSS (1977) *Joint Care Planning: health and local authorities* (London, DHSS Circular [HC(77)17, LAC(77)6]).

DHSS (1981) *Care in the Community: a consultative document on moving resources for care in England* (London, DHSS).

DHSS (1983a) *Explanatory Notes on Care in the Community* (London, DHSS).

DHSS (1983b) *Health Service development: care in the community and joint finance* (London, DHSS Circular [HC(83)6, LAC(83)5]).

DHSS (1983c) *NHS Management Enquiry* (Leader of Enquiry, Sir Roy Griffiths) (London, DHSS).

Disabled Persons (Services, Consultation and Representation) Act, 1986.

Doel, Mark and Peter Marsh (1992) *Task-Centred Social Work* (Aldershot, Hants, Ashgate).

DoE/DoH (1992) *Housing and Community Care* (London, DoE/DoH Circular [Department of the Environment 10/92, LAC(92)12]).

DoH (1989a) *Working for Patients* (CM555) (London, HMSO).

DoH (1989b) *Community Care in the Next Decade and Beyond* (London, HMSO).

DoH (1990) *Community Care in the Next Decade and Beyond: Policy Guidance* (London, HMSO).

DoH (1991) *Training for Community Care: a Joint Approach* (London, HMSO).

DoH (1992a) 'Care programming and mental health', *Caring for People* 10, pp. 11–12.

DoH (1992b) *Caring for People who Live at Home* (London, DoH [LASSL(92)7]).

DoH (1992c) *Implementing Caring for People* (London, DoH [EL(92)13; CI(92)10]).

DoH (1992d) *Community Care Special Transitional Grant* (London, DoH [EL(92)67; LASSL(92)8]).

DoH (1993a) *Community Care Plans (Consultation) Directions, 1993* (London, DoH [LAC(93)4]).

DoH (1993b) *Training for the Future: Training and Development Guidance to Support the Implementation of the NHS and Community Care Act 1990 and the Full Range of Community Care Reforms* (London, HMSO).

DoH (1993c) *Special Study: 31 December Agreements: Reviewing the implementation* (London, DoH).

DoH (1993d) *A Special Study of Purchasing and Contracting* (London, DoH).

DoH (1993e) *Community Care Monitoring: Special Study: Mental Health Services* (London, DoH).

DoH (1993f) *Implementing Community Care for Younger People with Physical and Sensory Disabilities: Report and findings of the SSI/NHSME special project* (London, DoH).

DoH (1994a) *Community Care Plans (Independent Sector Non-residential Care) Direction, 1994* (London, DoH [LAC(94)12]).

DoH (1994b) *Inspecting Social Services* (London, DoH [LAC(94)16]).

DoH/DSS (1993) *Independent Living Arrangements from April 1993* (London, DoH/DSS Circular [LASSL(93)6]).

DoH/SSI (1991) *Purchase of Service: Practice Guidance and Practice Material for Social Services Departments and Other Agencies* (London, HMSO).

DoH/Welsh Office (1993) *Code of Practice: Mental Health Act, 1983* (London, HMSO).

Emerson, Eric (1992) 'What is normalisation', in Hilary Brown and Helen Smith, *Normalisation: a reader for the nineties* (London, Tavistock/Routledge) pp. 1–18.

Felce, David (1993) 'Is community care expensive? The costs and benefits of residential models for people with severe mental handicap', *Mental Handicap*, 21, March, pp. 2–6.

Ferlie, Ewan, David Challis and Bleddyn Davies (1989) *Efficiency–Improving Innovations in Social Care of the Elderly* (Aldershot, Hants, Gower).

Fiedler, Barry (1993) *Getting Results: unlocking community care in partnership with disabled people* (London, King's Fund Centre) Living Options Partnership Paper 1.

Finch, Janet (1989) *Family Obligations and Social Change* (London, Polity).

Finch, Janet and Jennifer Mason (1993) *Negotiating Family Responsibilities* (London, Tavistock/Routledge).

Finkelstein, Vic (1990) 'From curing or caring to defining disabled people', in Jan Walmsley, Jill Reynolds, Pam Shakespeare and Ray Woolfe (1993) *Health Welfare and Practice: reflecting on roles and relationships* (London, Sage).

Firth Report (1987) *Public Support for Residential Care* (Report of a joint central and local government working party) (London, DHSS).

Fisher, Mike (1990a) 'Care management and social work: clients with dementia', *Practice*, 4(4), pp. 229–41.

Fisher, Mike (1990b) 'Care management and social work: working with carers', *Practice*, 4(4), pp. 242–52.

Fletcher, Peter (1993) 'Housing and community care: from rhetoric to reality', *Community Care Management and Planning*, 1(5), pp. 137–47.

Flynn, Norman (1993) 'Commentary on Contracting: a view from the voluntary sector', *Community Care Management and Planning* 1(4), pp. 114–15.

Flynn, Norman and Clive Miller (1991) *Caring in our Communities: the Management Agenda* (London, National Institute for Social Work Information Service).

Freire, Paulo (1972) *Pedagogy of the Oppressed* (Harmondsworth, Middlesex, Penguin).

Gilbert, Neil and Harry Specht (1976) 'Advocacy and professional ethics', *Social Work*, 21(4), pp. 288–93.

Glendinning, Caroline (1992) *The Costs of Informal Care: looking inside the household* (London, HMSO).

Goffman, Erving (1961) *Asylums: essays on the social situation of mental patients and other inmates* (Harmondsworth, Penguin).

Gomm, Richard, Alison Cathles Hagen, David Rudge and Randall Smith (1993) 'Whose need is it anyway? a care management project in Cheltenham', in Randall Smith, Lucy Gaster, Lynn Harrison, Linda Martin, Robin Means and Peter Thistlethwaite, *Working Together for Better Community Care* (Bristol, School for Advanced Urban Studies).

Goodwin, Simon (1989) 'Community care for the mentally ill in England and Wales: myths, assumptions and reality', *Journal of Social Policy*, 18(1), pp. 27–52.

Goodwin, Simon (1990) *Community Care and the Future of Mental Health Service Provision* (Aldershot, Hants, Avebury).

Gordon, Richard (1993) *Community Care Assessments: a practical legal framework* (London, Longman).

Graham, Hilary (1993), 'Feminist perspectives on caring', in Joanna Bornat, Charmaine Pereira, David Pilgrim and Fiona Williams, *Community Care: a reader* (London, Macmillan) pp. 124–33.

Grant, Gordon, Morag McGrath and Sheila Humphreys (eds) (1986) *Community Mental Handicap Teams: Theory and Practice* (Kidderminster, Worcs, British Institute of Mental Handicap).

Gray, Barbara (1989) *Collaborating: Finding Common Ground for Multiparty Problems* (San Francisco, CA, Jossey–Bass).

Griffiths, R. (Sir Roy) (1988) *Community Care: Agenda for Action* (The Griffiths Report) (London, HMSO).

Hadley, Roger and Stephen Hatch (1981) *Social Welfare and the Failure of the State* (London Allen & Unwin).

Hadley, R. and M. McGrath (eds) (1980) *Going Local – Neighbourhood Social Services* (London, Bedford Square Press).

Hadley, Roger and Morag McGrath (1984) *When Social Services are Local: the Normanton Experience* (London, Allen & Unwin).

Hadley, Roger and Ken Young (1990) *Creating a Responsive Public Service* (Hemel Heapstead, Harvester Wheatsheaf).

Hadley, Roger, Mike Cooper, Peter Dale and Graham Stacy (1987) *A Community Social Worker's Handbook* (London, Tavistock).

Hadley, Roger, Peter Dale and Patrick Sills (1984) *Decentralising Social Services: a model to change* (London, Bedford Square Press).

Haffenden, Sharon (1991) *Getting it Right for Carers: setting up services for carers: a guide for practitioners* (London, HMSO).

Haggard, Liz and Hester Ormiston (1993) 'Joint commissioning and joint working in South Derbyshire', *Community Care Management and Planning*, 1(3), pp. 77–85.

Hallett, Christine (1991) 'The Children Act, 1989 and Community Care: comparisons and contrasts', *Policy and Politics*, 19(4), pp. 283–91.

Ham, Chris, Ray Robinson and Michaela Benzeval (1990) *Health Check: health care reforms in an international context* (London, King's Fund Institute).

Harden, Ian (1992) *The Contracting State* (Buckingham, Open University Press).

Hardy, Brian, Gerald Wistow, and Ian Leedham (1993) *Analysis of a Sample of English Community Care Plans 1993/94* (London, Department of Health).

Harrison, Lyn and Peter Thistlethwaite (1993) 'Care management in a primary health care setting: pilot projects in East Sussex', in Randall Smith, Lucy Gaster, Lyn Harrison, Linda Martin, Robin Means and Peter Thistlethwaite, *Working Together for Better Community Care* (Bristol, School for Advanced Urban Studies).

Harrison, John (1987) *Severe Physical Disability: Responses to the Challenge of Care* (London, Cassell).

Hawley, Keith (nd, 1992?) *From Grants to Contracts: a Practical Guide for Voluntary Organisations* (London, Directory of Social Change/National Council for Voluntary Organisations).

Health Services and Public Health Act, 1968.

Heginbotham, Chris (1990) *Return to Community: the voluntary ethic and community care* (London, Bedford Square Press).

Henderson, Paul and Armstrong, John (1993) 'Community development and community care: a strategic approach', in Joanna Bornat, Charmaine Pereira, David Pilgrim and Fiona Williams, *Community Care: a reader* (London, Macmillan) pp. 156–63.

Henwood, Melanie and Malcolm Wicks (1985) 'Community care, family trends and social change', *Quarterly Journal of Social Affairs* 1(4), pp. 357–71.

Hills, Dionne (1991) *Carer Support in the Community: Evaluation of the*

Department of Health Initiative: 'Demonstration Districts for Informal Carers; 1986–1989' (London, HMSO).

Hounslow SSD (1992) *'First steps along the way . . .': the assessment pilot project in Feltham, Bedfont and Hanworth (older people and their carers)* (London, Hounslow Social Services Department Research and Development).

House of Commons Select Committee on the Social Services (1985) *Community Care: with special reference to adult mentally ill and mentally handicapped people* HC 13–1, 1984–5 (London, HMSO).

House of Commons Social Services Committee (1990) *Community Care: Carers* (London, HMSO).

Hoyes, Lesley and Marilyn Taylor (1993) 'Users' views on the community care reforms', *Community Care Management and Planning*, 1(3), pp. 87–90.

Hughes, Beverley (1993) 'A model for the comprehensive assessment of older people and their carers', *British Journal of Social Work*, 23(4), pp. 245–64.

Hunter, David (ed.) (1988) *Bridging the Gap: Case Management and Advocacy for People with Physical Handicaps* (London, King Edward's Hospital Fund for London).

Hunter, David (1994) 'The impact of the NHS reforms on community care', in Mike Titterton (ed.), *Caring for People in the Community: the new welfare* (London, Jessica Kingsley) pp. 12–23.

Hunter, David J. and Gerald Wistow (1987) *Community Care in Britain: variations on a theme* (London, King Edward's Hospital Fund for London).

Huxley, P. (1991) 'Effective case management for mentally ill people: the relevance of recent evidence from the USA for case management services in the United Kingdom', *Social Work and Social Services Review*, 2(3), pp. 192–203.

Huxley, Peter (1993), 'Case management and care management in community care', *British Journal of Social Work*, 23(4), pp. 365–81.

Jackson, Hilary and Simon Field (1989), *Race, Community Groups and Service Delivery* (London, HMSO).

Jamieson, Anne (1991) 'Community care for older people: policies in Britain, West Germany and Denmark', in Graham Room (ed.), *Towards a European Welfare State?* (Bristol, School for Advanced Urban Studies).

Jansen, Elly (ed.) (1980) *The Therapeutic Community Outside the Hospital* (London, Croom Helm).

Jays, Paul and Keith Bilton (1991) *Practising Care Management: the Gloucestershire Experience* (Gloucester: Gloucestershire County Council, Gloucestershire Family Health Services Authority, Cheltenham and District Health Authority, Gloucester Health Authority, CSL Group Limited).

Jones, Dee A. (1993) 'Informal carers and their elderly dependents: a community-based longitudinal study', in Diana Robbins (ed.), *Community Care: findings from Department of Health funded research 1988–1992* (London, HMSO) pp. 180–2.

Jones, Maxwell (1968) *Social Psychiatry in Practice* (Harmondsworth, Penguin).

Jordan, B. (1975) 'Is the client a fellow citizen?', *Social Work Today*, 6(15), pp. 471–5.

Kemshall, Hazel (1986) *Defining Clients' Needs in Social Work* (Norfolk, Norwich, Social Work Monographs).

Kennard, David (1983) *An Introduction to Therapeutic Communities* (London, Routledge).

Klein, Josephine (1965) *Samples from English Cultures, vol. 1* (London Routledge & Kegan Paul).

Knapp, Martin, Paul Cambridge, Corinne Thomason, Jennifer Beecham, Caroline Allen and Robin Darton (1990) *Care in the Community: lessons from a demonstration programme* (Canterbury, Kent, Personal Social Services Research Unit).

Knapp, Martin, Paul Cambridge, Corinne Thomason, Jennifer Beecham, Caroline Allen and Robin Darton (1992) *Care in the Community: challenge and demonstration* (Aldershot, Hants, Ashgate).

KPMG Management Consulting (1992) *Improving Independent Sector Involvement in Community Care Planning* (London, DoH).

KPMG Peat Marwick (1993) *Diversification and the Independent Residential Care Sector: a manual for residential care home providers* (London, HMSO).

Kroll, Robert J. and Ronald W. Stampfl (1981) 'The new consumerism', *Proceedings of the American Council on Consumer Interests*, 27th Annual Conference, April 1981, pp. 97–100.

Laczko, Frank and Chris Phillipson (1991) *Changing Work and Retirement* (Buckingham, Open University Press).

Land, Hilary (1988) 'Social security and community care: creating "perverse incentives"', in Sally Baldwin, Gillan Parker and Robert Walker (eds), *Social Security and Community Care* (Aldershot, Hants, Avebury).

Lawson, Alan (1993) *Assessment and Care Management Pilot Project: people with mental health problems* (London, Hounslow Social Services Department).

Lawson, Robyn (1993) 'The new technology of management in the personal social services', in Peter Taylor-Gooby and Robyn Lawson (eds), *Markets and Managers: new issues in the delivery of welfare* (Buckingham, Open University Press).

Leat, Diana (1983) 'Explaining volunteering: a sociological perspective', in Stephen Hatch (ed.), *Volunteers: patterns, meanings and motives* (Berkhamsted, Herts, The Volunteer Centre).

Leat, Diana and Pat Gay (1987) *Paying for Care: a study of policy and practice in paid care schemes* (London, Policy Studies Institute).

Leather, Philip and Sheila Mackintosh (1993) 'The long-term impact of staying put', *Ageing and Society*, 13, pp. 193–211.

Leritz, Len (1991) *No Fault Negotiating: How to Make Deals so that Both Sides Win* (Wellingborough, Northants, Thorsons).

Levin, Enid, Ian Sinclair, Peter Gorbach, Lorna Essame, Nori Graham, Jill Mortimer, Gillian Waldron and Jan Waterson (1989) *Families, Services and Confusion in Old Age* (Aldershot, Hants, Avebury).

Lewis, Jane (1993) 'Community care: policy imperatives, joint planning and enabling authorities', *Journal of Interprofessional Care*, 7(1), pp. 7–14.

Lewis, Sue (1993) 'Contracting: a view from the voluntary sector', *Community Care Management and Planning*, 1(4), pp. 108–14.

Local Authority Social Services Act, 1970.

Local Government Act, 1988.

Local Government Act, 1991.

Lynch, Bruce and Richard Perry (eds)(1992) *Experiences of Community Care: case studies of UK Practice* (London, Longman).

McGrath, Morag (1991) *Multi-disciplinary Teams* (Aldershot, Hants, Gower).

McGrath, Morag and Gordon Grant (1992) 'Supporting "needs-led" services: implications for planning and management systems (a case study in mental handicap services)', *Journal of Social Policy*, 21(1), pp. 71–98.

Maher, Janet and Oliver Russell (1988) 'Serving people with very challenging behaviour', in David Towell (ed.), *An Ordinary Life in Practice: developing comprehensive community-based services for people with learning disabilities* (London, King Edward's Hospital Fund for London).

Mansell Committee (1993) *Services for People with Learning Disabilities and Challenging Behaviour or Mental Health Needs: report of a project group* (London, HMSO).

Mansell, Jim and Fran Beasley (1993) 'Small staffed homes for people with a severe learning disability and challenging behaviour', *British Journal of Social Work*, 23(4), pp. 329–44.

Marsh, Peter and Mike Fisher (1992) *Good Intentions: developing partnership in social services* (York, Joseph Rowntree Foundation).

Mayo, Marjorie (1994) *Communities and Caring: the mixed economy of welfare* (London, Macmillan).

Meethan, Kevin and Catherine Thompson (1993) 'Politics, locality and resources: negotiating a community care scheme', *Policy and Politics*, 21(3), pp. 195–205.

Mental Health Act, 1959.

Meyer, Carol (1993) *Assessment in Social Work Practice* (New York, Columbia University Press).

Millard, David W. (1992) 'The therapeutic community in an age of community care', in Stephen R. Baron and J. Douglas Haldane, *Community, Normality and Difference: meeting special needs* (Aberdeen, Aberdeen University Press).

Miller, G. (1983) 'Case management: the essential service', in C. J. Sanborn (ed.), *Case Management in Mental Health Services* (New York, Haworth Press).

Morgan, Philip I. (1987) 'Resolving conflict through "win–win" negotiating', in Roy J. Lewicki, Joseph A. Litterer, David M. Saunders and John W. Minton (1993) *Negotiation: Readings, Exercises and Cases* (Homewood, Il, Irwin) pp. 125–9.

Morris, Jenny (1993a) '"Us" and "Them"? Feminist research and community care', in Joanna Bornat, Charmaine Pereira, David Pilgrim and Fiona Williams, *Community Care: a reader* (London, Macmillan) pp. 156–63.

Morris, Jenny (1993b) *Independent Lives: community care and disabled people* (London, Macmillan).

Moxley, David P. (1989) *The Practice of Case Management* (Beverly Hills, CA, Sage).

Murphy, Elaine (1991) *After the Asylums: community care for people with mental illness* (London, Faber & Faber).

National Health Service and Community Care Act, 1990.

Netten, Ann and Jennifer Beecham (eds)(1993) *Costing Community Care: Theory and Practice* (Aldershot, Hants, Ashgate).

Netten, Ann and Steve Smart (1993) *Unit Costs of Community Care 1992/ 1993* (Canterbury, Personal Social Services Research Unit).

Norman, Alison (1985) *Triple Jeopardy: growing old in a second homeland* (London, Centre for Policy on Ageing).

Obaze, David (1992) 'Black people and volunteering', in Rodney Hedley and Justin Davis Smith, *Volunteering and Society: principles and practice* (London, Bedford Square Press), pp. 132–43.

Oliver, Michael (1990) *The Politics of Disablement* (London, Macmillan).

Onyett, Steve and Sue Davenport (1993) 'Care programming and care management in Rochester', *Community Care Management and Planning*, 1(4), pp. 116–20.

Orbell, Sheina, Nicholas Hopkins and Brenda Gillies (1993) 'Measuring the impact of informal caring', *Journal of Community and Applied Social Psychology*, 3, pp. 149–63.

Orme, Joan and Brian Glastonbury (1994) *Care Management* (London, Macmillan).

Øvretveit, John (1993) *Co-ordinating Community Care: multidisciplinary teams and care management* (Buckingham, Open University Press).

Packman, Jean (1981) *The Child's Generation* (2nd edn) (Oxford, Basil Blackwell).

Parker, Gillian (1993a) *'With this Body': caring and disability in marriage* (Buckingham, Open University Press).

Parker, Gillian (1993b) 'Disability, caring and marriage the experience of young couples when a partner is disabled after marriage,' *British Journal of Social Work*, 23(6), pp. 565–80.

Parker, Gillian and Dot Lawton (1994) *Different Types of Care, Different Types of Carer: evidence from the General Household Survey* (London, HMSO).

Parker, Roy A. (1988) 'An historical background', in Ian Sinclair (ed.), *Residential Care: the research reviewed* (London, HMSO).

Parsloe, Phyllida (1986) 'What skills do social workers need?', in BASW *Skills for Social Workers in the 1980s* (Birmingham, BASW Publication).

Patmore, Charles (ed.) (1987) *Living After Mental Illness: innovations in services* (London, Croom Helm).

Patti, Rino J. (1971) 'Limitations and prospects of internal advocacy', *Social Casework*, 55(9), pp. 537–45.

Bibliography

247

Payne, Malcolm (1982) *Working in Teams* (London, Macmillan).

Payne, Malcolm (1986a) *Social Care in the Community* (London, Macmillan).

Payne, Malcolm (1986b) 'Implementing community social work from a social services department: some issues', *British Journal of Social Work*, 13(4), pp. 435–42.

Payne, Malcolm (1987) 'Prepare for a takeover bid now', *Community Care*, 8 January, p. 11.

Payne, Malcolm (1989) 'Open records and shared decisions with clients', in Steven Shardlow (ed.), *The Values of Change in Social Work* (London, Tavistock/Routledge).

Payne, Malcolm (1991) *Modern Social Work Theory: a Critical Introduction* (London, Macmillan).

Payne, Malcolm (1992) 'Psychodynamic theories within the politics of social work theory', *Journal of Social Work Practice*, 6(2), pp. 141–9.

Payne, Malcolm (1993a) *Linkages: effective networking in social care* (London, Whiting & Birch).

Payne, Malcolm (1993b) 'Routes to and through clienthood and their implications for practice', *Practice*, 6(3), pp. 169–80.

Payne, Malcolm (1993c) 'New understandings of Later Life: practice and service implications' in Peter R. Day (ed.), *Perspectives on Later Life* (London, Whiting & Birch) pp. 1–21.

Percy Report (1957) *Report of the Royal Commission on the Law Relating to Mental Illness and Mental Deficiency* (Cmnd 169) (London, HMSO).

Perring, Christine, Julia Twigg and Karl Atkin (1990) *Families Caring for People Diagnosed as Mentally Ill: the literature re-examined* (London, HMSO).

Petch, Alison (1994) '"The best move I've made": the role of housing for those with mental health problems', in Mike Titterton (ed.), *Caring for People in the Community: the new welfare* (London, Jessica Kingsley) pp. 76–90.

Pfeffer, Naomi and Anna Coote (1991) *Is Quality Good for You? a critical review of quality assurance in welfare services* (London, Institute for Public Policy Research).

Philp, Mark (1979) 'Notes on the form of knowledge in social work', *Sociological Review*, 27(1), pp. 83–111.

Pilling, Doria (1992) *Approaches to Case Management for People with Disabilities* (London, Jessica Kingsley).

Pilling, Stephen (1991) *Rehabilitation and Community Care* (London, Routledge).

Pinch, Helen (1993) 'The barriers to homeless people accessing community care', *Community Care Management and Planning* 5(1), pp. 131–5.

Platt, Stephen, with Rite Piepe and Judith Smyth (1988) *Teams: a game to develop group skills* (Aldershot, Hants, Gower).

Positive Publications (1993) *Fit for the Community: a practical guide to care management and community care of people with mental health problems* (London, Positive Publications).

Potter, John (1988) 'Consumerism and the public sector: how well does the coat fit?', *Public Administration*, 66(2), pp. 149–64.

Poynter, Richard and Clive Martin (1994) *Rights Guide to Non-Means-Tested Benefits* (London, Child Poverty Action Group).

Presland, Tom (1990) *Volunteers and Community Care* (Berkhamsted, Herts, The Volunteer Centre UK).

Price Waterhouse/DoH (1993) *Implementing Community Care: Population Needs Assessment Good Practice Guide* (London, Department of Health).

Pruitt, Dean G. and Peter J. Carnevale (1993) *Negotiation in Social Conflict* (Buckingham, Open University Press).

Pruitt, Dean and Jeffrey Rubin (1986) *Social Conflict* (New York, McGraw-Hill).

Putnam, Linda L. and Michael E. Roloff (1992) *Communication and Negotiation* (Newbury Park, CA, Sage).

Qureshi, Hazel, David Challis and Bleddyn Davies (1989) *Helpers in Case-Managed Community Care* (Aldershot, Hants, Gower).

Raiff, Norma Radol and Barbara K. Shore (1993) *Advanced Case Management: New strategies for the nineties* (Newbury Park, CA, Sage).

Ramon, Shulamit (1988) 'Towards normalization: polarization and change in Britain', in Shulamit Ramon and Maria Grazia Giannichedda (1988) *Psychiatry in Transition: the British and Italian experiences* (London, Pluto) pp. 261–72.

Ramon, Shulamit (ed.) (1991) *Beyond Community Care: normalisation and integration work* (London, Macmillan).

Ramon, Shulamit and Maria Grazia Giannichedda (1988) *Psychiatry in Transition: the British and Italian experiences* (London, Pluto).

Reading, Paul (nd, 1994?) *Community Care and the Voluntary Sector: the role of voluntary organisations in a changing world* (Birmingham, Venture).

Rees, Stuart (1991) *Achieving Power: Practice and Policy in Social Welfare* (Sydney, Allen & Unwin).

Renshaw, J. (1988) 'Care in the community: individual care planning and case management', in B. Davies and M. Knapp (eds), *The Production of Welfare Approach: evidence and argument from the PSSRU*, Supplement to the *British Journal of Social Work*, 18, pp. 70–106.

Renshaw, J., R. Hampson, C. Thomason, R. Darton, K. Judge and M. Knapp (1989) *Care in the Community: the first steps* (Aldershot, Hants, Gower).

Richardson, Ann and Jane Ritchie (1989) *Developing Friendships: enabling people with learning difficulties to make and maintain friends* (London, Policy Studies Institute).

Richardson, Ann, Judith Unell and Beverly Aston (1989) *A New Deal for Carers* (London, Kings Fund Informal Caring Programme).

Righton, Peter (ed.) (1979) *Studies in Environment Therapy vol. 3* (Toddington, Glos, Planned Environment Therapy Trust).

Riley, Christopher (1993) 'Community services in Wales towards 2010', *Community Care Management and Planning*, 1(3), pp. 67–75.

Ritchie Report (1994) *The Report of the Inquiry into the Care and Treatment of Christopher Clumis* (London, HMSO).

Robbins, Diana (ed.) (1993) *Community Care: Findings from Department of Health Funded Research 1988–1992* (London, HMSO).

Robinson, Carol (1991) *Home and Away: respite care in the community* (Birmingham, Venture).

Robinson, Janice and Lydia Yee (1991) *Focus on Carers: a practical guide to planning and delivering community care services* (London, King's Fund Centre).

Rochester, Colin (1992) 'Community organisations and voluntary action', in Rodney Hedley and Justin Davis Smith, *Volunteering and Society: principles and practice* (London, Bedford Square Press) pp. 120–31.

Rose, Stephen M. and Bruce L. Black (1985) *Advocacy and Empowerment: mental health care in the community* (Boston, Routledge & Kegan Paul).

Royston, Stephen and Lisa Rodrigues (1993) 'Integrated assessment in East Sussex', *Community Care Management and Planning*, 1(2), pp. 35–43.

Schneider, Justine (1993) 'Care programming in mental health: assimilation and adaptation', *British Journal of Social Work*, 23(4), pp. 383–403.

Schorr, Alvin, L. (1992) *The Personal Social Services: an outside view* (York, Joseph Rowntree Foundation).

Seebohm Report (1968) *Report of the Committee on Local Authority and Allied Personal Social Services* (Cmnd 3703) (London, HMSO).

Seed, Philip (1990) *Introducing Network Analysis in Social Work* (London, Jessica Kingsley).

Sherlock, Jan (1991) *At Home in the Community: a directory of housing and support services for people in long-term contact with mental health agencies* (London, Good Practices in Mental Health).

Sherrott, Roger (1983) 'Fifty volunteers', in Stephen Hatch (ed.), *Volunteers: patterns, meanings and motives* (Berkhamsted, Herts, The Volunteer Centre).

Simic, Paul (1994) 'Moving out of hospital into the community', in Mike Titterton (ed.), *Caring for People in the Community: the new welfare* (London, Jessica Kingsley) pp. 55–75.

Sinclair, Elma (1988) 'Guide to the evidence (ii) The formal evidence', in National Institute for Social Work, *Residential Care: a positive choice* (Report of the Independent Review of Residential Care chaired by Gillan Wagner) (London, HMSO) Appendix 1, pp. 161–224.

Sinclair, Ian, David Crosbie, Pat O'Connor, Lorraine Stanforth and Anne Vickery (1988) *Bridging Two Worlds: social work and the elderly living alone* (Aldershot, Hants, Gower).

Sinclair, Ian, Roy Parker, Diana Leat and Jenny Williams (1990) *The Kaleidoscope of Care: a review of research on welfare provision for elderly people* (London, HMSO).

Smale, Gerald and William Bennett (1989) *Pictures of Practice: vol. 1 Community Social Work in Scotland* (London, National Institute for Social Work).

Smale, Gerald, and Graham Tuson (1990) 'Community social work: foundation for the 1990s and beyond', in Giles Darvill and Gerald Smale (eds), *Partners in Empowerment: networks of innovation in social work* (London, National Institute for Social Work).

Smale, Gerald, Graham Tuson, Nina Biehal and Peter Marsh (1993) *Empowerment, Assessment, Care Management and the Skilled Worker* (London, HMSO).

Smale, Gerald, Graham Tuson, Mike Cooper, Mike Wardle and David Crosbie (1988) *Community Social Work: a paradigm for change* (London, National Institute for Social Work).

Smith, Gilbert (1980) *Social Need: Policy, Practice and Research* (London, Routledge & Kegan Paul).

Smith, Helen (1992) 'Links between case management and contracting' in Edward Peck, Peter Ritchie and Helen Smith, *Contracting and Case Management in Community Care: the challenges for local authorities* (London, CCETSW, Paper 32).

Smith, Randall, Lucy Gaster, Lynn Harrison, Linda Martin, Robin Means and Peter Thistlethwaite, (1993) *Working Together for Better Community Care* (Bristol, School for Advanced Urban Studies).

Solomon, Barbara B. (1976) *Black Empowerment* (New York, Columbia University Press).

Solomon, Barbara Bryant (1989) 'How do we really empower families? New strategies for social work practitioners' in Beulah R. Compton and Burt Galaway, *Social Work Processes* (4th edn) (Belmont, CA, Wadsworth) pp. 529–32.

SSI (1991a), *The Right to Complain: practice guidance on complaints procedures in social services departments* (London, HMSO).

SSI (1991b) *Complaints about the Social Services Department: ideas for a practice booklet for clerks, receptionists and telephonists* (London, HMSO).

SSI (1991c) *Getting the Message Across: a Guide to Developing and Communicating Policies, Principles and Procedures on Assessment* (London, HMSO).

SSI (1993) *Mental Illness Specific Grant: second report on monitoring its use 1991/2* (London, HMSO).

SSI/NHSME (1993) *Assessment Special Study: a joint SSI/NHSME study of assessment procedures in five local authority areas* (London, DoH).

SSI/RHA (1993) *SSI/RHA Community Care Monitoring September 1993: national summary* (London, DoH).

SSI/SWSG (1991a) *Care Management and Assessment: Practitioners' Guide* (London, DoH SSI/SWSG).

SSI/SWSG (1991b) *Care Management and Assessment: Managers' Guide* (London, DoHSSI/SWSG).

SSI/SWSG (1991c) *Care Management and Assessment: Summary of Practice Guidance* (London, DoHSSI/SWSG).

Stace, Sheila and Jane Tunstill (1990) *On Different Tracks: the inconsistencies between the Children Act and the Community Care Act* (London, VOPSS).

Stacey, Margaret (1969) 'The myth of community studes', *British Journal of Sociology*, 20(2), pp. 134–47.

Stalker, Karen (1993) 'The efficiency and effectiveness of community care: evaluation of pilot projects: (1) Tayside Region', in Social Work Research Centre, Stirling, *Is Social Work Effective? Research findings from the Social Work Research Centre* (Stirling, Social Work Research Centre).

Steinberg, R. M. and G. W. Carter (1983) *Case Management and the Elderly* (Lexington Books).

Stevenson, Olive and Phyllida Parsloe (1993) *Community Care and Empowerment* (York, Joseph Rowntree Foundation).

Stuart, R. (1964) 'Supportive casework with borderline patients', *Social Work*, 9(1), pp. 38–44.

Szivos, Sue (1992) 'The limits to integration?', in Hilary Brown and Helen Smith, *Normalisation: a reader for the nineties* (London, Routledge).

Taylor, Brian and Toni Devine (1993) *Assessing Needs and Planning Care in Social Work* (Aldershot, Hants, Arena).

Taylor, Cathy (1993) 'An evaluation of a multi-disciplinary pilot project "Assessment of Social Care Needs" for elderly people in Borders Region', in Social Work Research Centre, Stirling, *Is Social Work Effective? Research findings from the Social Work Research Centre* (Stirling, Social Work Research Centre).

Taylor, Max and Christine Vigars (1993) *Management and Delivery of Social Care* (London, Longman).

Thompson, Neil (1993) *Anti-discriminatory Practice* (London, Macmillan).

Thompson, P. (1992) 'Community care – so what's new?', *Welfare Rights Bulletin*, 112 (February 1992), pp. 6–9.

Tomlinson, Dylan Ronald (1991) *Utopia, Community Care and the Retreat from the Asylums* (Milton Keynes, Open University Press).

Tönnies, F. (1955) *Community and Association* (London, Routledge & Kegan Paul).

Towell, David (ed.) (1988) *An Ordinary Life in Practice* (London, King Edward's Hospital Fund for London).

Townsend, Peter (1962) *The Last Refuge: a survey of residential institutions and homes for the aged in England and Wales* (London, Routledge & Kegan Paul).

Twigg, Julia, Karl Atkin and Christina Perring (1990) *Carers and Services: a review of research* (London, HMSO).

Wagner Report (1988) *Residential. Care: a positive choice* (Report of the Independent Review of Residential Care) (London, HMSO).

Walsh, Kieron (1989) 'Contract Management: a new role for local government', in Isobel Allen (ed.), *Social Services Departments as Managing Agencies* (London, Policy Studies Institute).

Walton, Ronald (ed.) (1986) 'Integrating formal and informal care: the utilization of social support networks', *British Journal of Social Work* vol. 16, supplement, pp. 1–179.

Warburton, William (1993) 'Performance indicators: what was all the fuss about?', *Community Care Management and Planning*, 1(4), pp. 99–105.

Weil, Marie (1985) 'Key components in providing efficient and effective services', in Marie Weil *et al*, *Case Management in Human Service*

Practice: a systematic approach to mobilising resources for clients (San Francisco, Jossey–Bass).

Weil, Marie and James M. Karls (1985) 'Historical origins and recent developments' in Marie Weil *et al* (1985) *Case Management in Human Service Practice: a systematic approach to mobilising resources for clients* (San Francisco, Jossey–Bass).

Weil, Marie, James M. Karls and Associates (1985) *Case Management in Human Service Practice: a systematic approach to mobilising resources for clients* (San Francisco, Jossey–Bass).

Weinstein, Jenny (1994) *Sewing the Seams for a Seamless Service: a review of development in interprofessional education and training* (London, CCETSW).

Weller, Malcolm P. I. and Mattijs Muijen (eds) (1993) *Dimensions of Community Mental Health Care* (London, W. B. Saunders).

Wenger, G. Clare (1994) *Understanding Support Networks and Community Care: network assessment for elderly people* (Aldershot, Hants, Avebury).

Williams, Paul and Alan Tyne (1988) 'Exploring values as the basis of service development' in David Towell (ed.), *An Ordinary Life in Practice: developing comprehensive community-based services for people with learning disabilities* (London, King Edward's Hospital Fund for London).

Williams, Raymond (1983) *Keywords: a vocabulary of culture and society* (London, Fontana).

Willis, Elaine (1992) 'Volunteers as advocates: some perspectives for the 1990s', in Rodney Hedley and Justin Davis Smith, *Volunteering and Society: principles and practice* (London, Bedford Square Press), pp. 144–54.

Willmott, Peter (1986) *Social Networks, Informal Care and Public Policy* (London, Policy Studies Institute).

Willmott, Peter (1989) *Community Initiatives: Patterns and Prospects* (London, Policy Studies Institute).

Wistow, Gerald (1982) 'Collaboration between health and local authorities: why is it necessary?', *Social Policy and Administration*, 16(1), pp. 44–62.

Wistow, Gerald, Ian Leedham and Brian Hardy (1993) *Community Care Plans: a preliminary sample of English Community Care Plans* (London, DoH/SSI).

Wolfensberger, Wolf (1972) *The Principle of Normalisation in Human Services* (Toronto: National Institute on Mental Retardation).

Wolfensberger, Wolf (1984) 'A reconceptualization of normalisation as social role valorization', *Mental Retardation*, 34, pp. 22–5.

Woolf, Jo (1992) *Beginner's Guide to Contracts* (London, London Voluntary Service Council).

Name Index

Subject Index

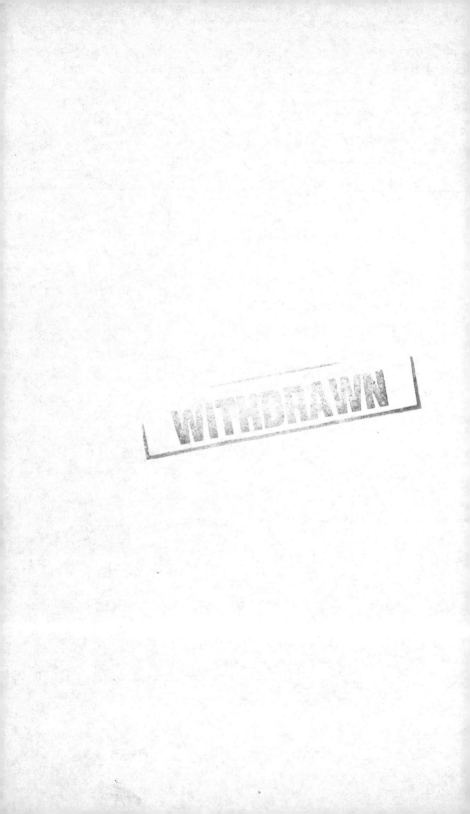